SYSTEMATIZING THE ONE HEALTH APPROACH IN PREPAREDNESS AND RESPONSE EFFORTS FOR INFECTIOUS DISEASE OUTBREAKS

PROCEEDINGS OF A WORKSHOP

Claire Biffl, Julie Liao, Charles Minicucci, and Anna Nicholson,
Rapporteurs

Forum on Microbial Threats

Board on Global Health

Health and Medicine Division

The National Academies of
SCIENCES • ENGINEERING • MEDICINE

THE NATIONAL ACADEMIES PRESS
Washington, DC
www.nap.edu

THE NATIONAL ACADEMIES PRESS   500 Fifth Street, NW   Washington, DC 20001

This activity was supported by contracts between the National Academy of Sciences and the Burroughs Wellcome Fund (#1021631), the New Venture Fund (#NVF-NGDF-NAT10-Subgrant-013445-2021-01-01), the U.S. Agency for International Development (#7200AA18GR00003), the U.S. Department of Defense (#HU0012110002), the U.S. Department of Health and Human Services (#75A50119C00031, #75D301-20-Q-71879, #R13FD006897, #HHSN263201800029I/HHSN26300011), the U.S. Department of Homeland Security (#70RSAT21G00000003), and the U.S. Department of Veterans Affairs (#VA250-16-C-0012/36C2501P2314). Any opinions, findings, conclusions, or recommendations expressed in this publication do not necessarily reflect the views of any organization or agency that provided support for the project.

International Standard Book Number-13: 978-0-309-09337-8
International Standard Book Number-10: 0-309-09337-6
Digital Object Identifier: https://doi.org/10.17226/26301

Additional copies of this publication are available from the National Academies Press, 500 Fifth Street, NW, Keck 360, Washington, DC 20001; (800) 624-6242 or (202) 334-3313; http://www.nap.edu.

Copyright 2022 by the National Academy of Sciences. All rights reserved.

Printed in the United States of America

Suggested citation: National Academies of Sciences, Engineering, and Medicine. 2022. *Systematizing the One Health approach in preparedness and response efforts for infectious disease outbreaks: Proceedings of a workshop*. Washington, DC: The National Academies Press. https://doi.org/10.17226/26301.

The National Academies of
SCIENCES · ENGINEERING · MEDICINE

The **National Academy of Sciences** was established in 1863 by an Act of Congress, signed by President Lincoln, as a private, nongovernmental institution to advise the nation on issues related to science and technology. Members are elected by their peers for outstanding contributions to research. Dr. Marcia McNutt is president.

The **National Academy of Engineering** was established in 1964 under the charter of the National Academy of Sciences to bring the practices of engineering to advising the nation. Members are elected by their peers for extraordinary contributions to engineering. Dr. John L. Anderson is president.

The **National Academy of Medicine** (formerly the Institute of Medicine) was established in 1970 under the charter of the National Academy of Sciences to advise the nation on medical and health issues. Members are elected by their peers for distinguished contributions to medicine and health. Dr. Victor J. Dzau is president.

The three Academies work together as the **National Academies of Sciences, Engineering, and Medicine** to provide independent, objective analysis and advice to the nation and conduct other activities to solve complex problems and inform public policy decisions. The National Academies also encourage education and research, recognize outstanding contributions to knowledge, and increase public understanding in matters of science, engineering, and medicine.

Learn more about the National Academies of Sciences, Engineering, and Medicine at **www.nationalacademies.org**.

The National Academies of
SCIENCES • ENGINEERING • MEDICINE

Consensus Study Reports published by the National Academies of Sciences, Engineering, and Medicine document the evidence-based consensus on the study's statement of task by an authoring committee of experts. Reports typically include findings, conclusions, and recommendations based on information gathered by the committee and the committee's deliberations. Each report has been subjected to a rigorous and independent peer-review process and it represents the position of the National Academies on the statement of task.

Proceedings published by the National Academies of Sciences, Engineering, and Medicine chronicle the presentations and discussions at a workshop, symposium, or other event convened by the National Academies. The statements and opinions contained in proceedings are those of the participants and are not endorsed by other participants, the planning committee, or the National Academies.

For information about other products and activities of the National Academies, please visit www.nationalacademies.org/about/whatwedo.

PLANNING COMMITTEE ON SYSTEMATIZING THE ONE HEALTH APPROACH IN PREPAREDNESS AND RESPONSE EFFORTS FOR INFECTIOUS DISEASE OUTBREAKS[1]

CASEY BARTON-BEHRAVESH (*Co-Chair*), Director, One Health Office, U.S. Centers for Disease Control
JONNA A. K. MAZET (*Co-Chair*), Professor of Epidemiology and Disease Ecology, School of Veterinary Medicine; Executive Director, One Health Institute, University of California, Davis
KEVIN ANDERSON, Senior Program Manager, Science and Technology Directorate, U.S. Department of Homeland Security
ANDREW CLEMENTS, Deputy Director, Pandemic Influenza and Other Emerging Threats Unit, U.S. Agency for International Development
PETER DASZAK, President, EcoHealth Alliance
EVA HARRIS, Professor, Division of Infectious Diseases and Vaccinology; Director, Center for Global Public Health, University of California, Berkeley
KENT KESTER, Vice President and Head, Translational Science and Biomarkers, Sanofi Pasteur
MAUREEN LICHTVELD, Dean, Graduate School of Public Health, Jonas Salk Professor of Population Health, Professor of Environmental and Occupational Health, University of Pittsburgh
SALLY A. MILLER, Distinguished Professor of Food, Agricultural and Environmental Sciences, Department of Plant Pathology, The Ohio State University
BRIANNA SKINNER, Senior Regulatory Veterinarian, Office of Counterterrorism and Emerging Threats, Office of the Chief Scientist, U.S. Food and Drug Administration
MARK S. SMOLINSKI, President, Ending Pandemics
MARY E. WILSON, Clinical Professor of Epidemiology & Biostatistics, School of Medicine, University of California, San Francisco

---

[1] The National Academies of Sciences, Engineering, and Medicine's planning committees are solely responsible for organizing the workshop, identifying topics, and choosing speakers. The responsibility for the published Proceedings of a Workshop rests with the workshop rapporteurs and the institution.

FORUM ON MICROBIAL THREATS[1]

PETER DASZAK (*Chair*), President, EcoHealth Alliance
KENT E. KESTER (*Vice Chair*), Vice President and Head, Translational Science and Biomarkers, Sanofi Pasteur
RIMA F. KHABBAZ (*Vice Chair*), Director, National Center for Emerging Zoonotic Infectious Diseases, U.S. Centers for Disease Control and Prevention
EMILY ABRAHAM, Director, External Affairs and Policy, Johnson & Johnson Global Public Health
KEVIN ANDERSON, Senior Program Manager, Science and Technology Directorate, U.S. Department of Homeland Security
CRISTINA CASSETTI, Deputy Division Director, Division of Microbiology and Infectious Diseases, National Institute of Allergy and Infectious Diseases, National Institutes of Health
ANDREW CLEMENTS, Senior Technical Advisor, Emerging Threats Division, U.S. Agency for International Development
SCOTT F. DOWELL, Deputy Director, Surveillance and Epidemiology, Bill & Melinda Gates Foundation
MARCOS A. ESPINAL, Director, Communicable Diseases and Health Analysis, Pan American Health Organization
EVA HARRIS, Professor, Division of Infectious Diseases and Vaccinology; Director, Center for Global Public Health, University of California, Berkeley
ELIZABETH D. HERMSEN, Head, Global Antimicrobial Stewardship and Health Equity in Infectious Disease, Merck & Co., Inc.
CHRISTOPHER HOUCHENS, Director, Division of Chemical, Biological, Radiological and Nuclear Countermeasures, Biomedical Advanced Research and Development Authority, U.S. Department of Health and Human Services
CHANDY C. JOHN, Director, Ryan White Center for Pediatric Infectious Disease and Global Health, Indiana University School of Medicine
MARK G. KORTEPETER, Vice President for Research, Uniformed Services University of the Health Sciences
MICHAEL MAIR, Acting Director, Office of Counterterrorism and Emerging Threats, U.S. Food and Drug Administration

---

[1] The National Academies of Sciences, Engineering, and Medicine's forums and roundtables do not issue, review, or approve individual documents. The responsibility for the published Proceedings of a Workshop rests with the workshop rapporteurs and the institution.

JONNA A. K. MAZET, Distinguished Professor of Epidemiology and Disease Ecology; Founding Executive Director, One Health Institute, University of California, Davis
VICTORIA McGOVERN, Senior Program Officer, Burroughs Wellcome Fund
SALLY A. MILLER, Distinguished Professor of Food, Agricultural and Environmental Sciences, The Ohio State University
SUERIE MOON, Director of Research, Global Health Centre; Visiting Lecturer, Graduate Institute of International and Development Studies, Geneva; Adjunct Lecturer, Harvard T.H. Chan School of Public Health
RAFAEL OBREGON, Chief of Communication for Development, United Nations Children's Fund
KUMANAN RASANATHAN, Health Systems Coordinator, Office of the WHO Representative in Cambodia, World Health Organization
GARY A. ROSELLE, Chief of Medical Service, Veterans Affairs Medical Center; Director, National Infectious Disease Services, Veterans Health Administration; U.S. Department of Veterans Affairs
PETER A. SANDS, Executive Director, The Global Fund to Fight AIDS, Tuberculosis and Malaria
THOMAS W. SCOTT, Distinguished Professor of Entomology and Nematology, University of California, Davis
MATTHEW ZAHN, Medical Director, Division of Epidemiology and Assessment, Orange County Health Care Agency

National Academies of Sciences, Engineering, and Medicine Staff

JULIE LIAO, Associate Program Officer *(from August 2020)*
CHARLES MINICUCCI, Research Assistant *(from July 2020)*
CLAIRE BIFFL, Senior Program Assistant *(from March 2021)*
JULIE PAVLIN, Director, Forum on Microbial Threats; Senior Director, Board on Global Health

Reviewers

This Proceedings of a Workshop was reviewed in draft form by individuals chosen for their diverse perspectives and technical expertise. The purpose of this independent review is to provide candid and critical comments that will assist the National Academies of Sciences, Engineering, and Medicine in making each published proceedings as sound as possible and to ensure that it meets the institutional standards for quality, objectivity, evidence, and responsiveness to the charge. The review comments and draft manuscript remain confidential to protect the integrity of the process.

We thank the following individuals for their review of this proceedings:

A. ALONSO AGUIRRE, George Mason University
LINDA A. McMAULEY, Emory University
ELIZABETH MUMFORD, World Health Organization

Although the reviewers listed above provided many constructive comments and suggestions, they were not asked to endorse the content of the proceedings nor did they see the final draft before its release. The review of this proceedings was overseen by **M. KARIUKI NJENGA,** Washington State University. He was responsible for making certain that an independent examination of this proceedings was carried out in accordance with standards of the National Academies and that all review comments were carefully considered. Responsibility for the final content rests entirely with the rapporteurs and the National Academies.

Contents

ACRONYMS AND ABBREVIATIONS   xv

1   INTRODUCTION   1
     Organization of the Proceedings of the Workshop, 2

2   KEYNOTE: ONE HEALTH AND PREVENTING
     PANDEMICS   7
     The One Health Approach, 7
     One Health Pandemic Response Framework, 9
     Global Interconnectedness, 14
     Discussion, 14

3   ONE HEALTH IN PRAXIS   19
     Operationalizing One Health at a Local Level, 20
     Multi-Sectoral Engagement in the COVID-19 Outbreak
        Response in Thailand, 25
     COVID-19 Response: Lessons Learned to Reinforce the
        Relevance of One Health Principles, 29
     Discussion, 35
     Reflections from Day 1, 39

4   CURRENT ONE HEALTH EFFORTS AND OPPORTUNITIES   43
     What Is Being Done Now?, 43
     Opportunities for Improvement, 55

5	**BUILDING THE FUTURE ONE HEALTH WORKFORCE**	65

The One Health Workforce: Reconciling Competencies with Opportunities, 65
University Networks on the Front Lines for Community Engagement and One Health Innovation, 71
Discussion, 75
Reflections on Day 2, 80

6	**LEARNING FROM THE PAST AND PLANNING FOR THE FUTURE OF ONE HEALTH**	83

Precision Epidemiology, Human Behavior, and the Future of One Health, 84
Collaborative Effort in Outbreak Preparedness: FDA's Approach to ASF, 88
Paradox of Global Policies for Pandemic Prediction and Prevention, 93
Taking Pandemic Threats Off the Table, 98
Discussion, 102

7	**BUILDING A BETTER SYSTEM FOR OUTBREAK RESPONSE, SURVEILLANCE, DETECTION, AND FORECASTING**	109

Breakout Session Highlights, 109
Discussion, 114

REFERENCES 121

APPENDIXES
A Workshop Statement of Task 127
B Workshop Agenda 129
C Speaker and Moderator Biographies 137

Boxes and Figures

BOXES

3-1 Fast-Tracked COVID-19 Emergency Management Efforts in Rwanda, 32
3-2 Lessons Learned from Rwanda's COVID-19 Response, 35

4-1 Data to Support the One Health Approach, 62

5-1 Uganda Students One Health Innovations Club, 74

7-1 Highlights from Discussion on Response Capacities, 110
7-2 Highlights from Discussion on Surveillance and Detection Mechanisms, 111
7-3 Highlights from Discussion on Forecasting and Predictive Innovations, 113

FIGURES

3-1 Harris County Public Health Department's response to West Nile Virus: Before and after the One Health approach, 22

6-1 Critical actions and response actors involved in outbreak containment, 87

Acronyms and Abbreviations

ACE-2　　　　angiotensin converting enzyme-2
Africa CDC　Africa Centres for Disease Control and Prevention
AFROHUN　Africa One Health University Network
ALERRT　　African coaLition for Epidemic Research, Response, and Training
AMR　　　　antimicrobial resistance
ASF　　　　African swine fever

BARDA　　　U.S. Biomedical Advanced Research and Development Authority

CDC　　　　U.S. Centers for Disease Control and Prevention
CEPI　　　　Coalition for Epidemic Preparedness Innovations
COVID-19　coronavirus disease 2019
CVM　　　　Center for Veterinary Medicine

DART　　　　during-action review and tabletop
DCCP　　　Disease Control and Clinical Prevention
DDC　　　　Department of Disease Control
DMSc　　　Department of Medical Science
DNP　　　　Department of National Parks, Wildlife, and Plant Conservation
DOD　　　　U.S. Department of Defense

EPH　　　　Environmental Public Health

EPI	epidemiology
FAO	Food and Agriculture Organization of the United Nations
FDA	U.S. Food and Drug Administration
GDP	gross domestic product
GHSA	Global Health Security Agenda
HCPH	Harris County Public Health
HIV	human immunodeficiency virus
IAR	intra-action review
IFTF	Institute for the Future
IHR	International Health Regulations
IMF	International Monetary Fund
IPBES	Intergovernmental Science-Policy Platform on Biodiversity and Ecosystem Services
IPE	interprofessional practice and education
MERS	Middle East respiratory syndrome
MOH	Ministry of Health
mRNA	messenger ribonucleic acid
MVCD	Mosquito and Vector Control Division
NIEHS	National Institute of Environmental Health Sciences
OHW-NG	One Health Workforce—Next Generation
OIE	World Organisation for Animal Health
PCR	polymerase chain reaction
PREP	Portal for Readiness Exercises and Planning
ProMED	Program for Monitoring Emerging Diseases
PVS	Performance of Veterinary Services Pathway
RBD	receptor binding domain
RT-PCR	reverse transcription polymerase chain reaction
SARS	severe acute respiratory syndrome
SARS-CoV-2	severe acute respiratory syndrome coronavirus 2
SEAOHUN	Southeast Asia One Health University Network
SOHIC	Students One Health Innovations Club
TB	tuberculosis

TRC-EID	Thai Red Cross Emerging Infectious Diseases Health Science Centre
UC Davis	University of California, Davis
UHC	universal health coverage
UN	United Nations
USAID	U.S. Agency for International Development
USDA	U.S. Department of Agriculture
VPH	Veterinary Public Health
WHO	World Health Organization
WTO	World Trade Organization

1

Introduction

On February 23–25, 2021, a planning committee convened by the Forum on Microbial Threats at the National Academies of Sciences, Engineering, and Medicine (the National Academies) held a 3-day virtual workshop titled Systematizing the One Health Approach in Preparedness and Response Efforts for Infectious Disease Outbreaks.[1] The workshop gave particular consideration to research opportunities, multisectoral collaboration mechanisms, community-engagement strategies, educational opportunities, and policies that speakers have found effective in implementing the core capacities and interventions of One Health principles to strengthen national health systems and enhance global health security. It featured presentations on the following topics:[2]

- Strategies to systematize One Health in national prevention, detection, preparedness, and response efforts;
- A review of One Health programs integrated into national and global public health efforts to learn what programs are currently in effect;

---

[1] The National Academies of Sciences, Engineering, and Medicine's planning committees are solely responsible for organizing the workshop, identifying topics, and choosing speakers. The responsibility for the published Proceedings of a Workshop rests with the workshop rapporteurs and the institution.

[2] The full Statement of Task is available in Appendix A.

- Integration of animal and human health surveillance systems for cross-reporting to better understand pathogens transmitted between animals and people;
- Feasibility of introducing and integrating One Health into existing coordination mechanisms and into national action plans for health security based on the Joint External Evaluation;[3]
- Strengthening the global health workforce with One Health capacities;
- Policies that underscore the interconnectedness of animal, plant, human, and environmental/ecosystem health;
- Implications of using a One Health approach to improve preparedness versus a reactive response that is required to apply medical countermeasures after the onset of an outbreak;
- Promising practices for engaging with communities and influencing behaviors that lower the risk of infectious disease through the One Health approach;
- The tension between public health needs, the private sector, and data sharing within the One Health context in preparedness and response efforts; and
- Potential priority actions to unite organizations—public and private, domestic and international—in efforts to overcome newly discovered hurdles based on lessons learned from the COVID-19 pandemic.

ORGANIZATION OF THE PROCEEDINGS OF THE WORKSHOP

In accordance with National Academies policies, the workshop did not attempt to establish any conclusions or recommendations about needs and future directions, focusing instead on information presented, questions raised, and improvements suggested by individual participants. Chapter 2 presents the workshop's keynote address, which outlined the One Health concept, gaps in current pandemic surveillance and response efforts, and strategies for continued integration of this approach into practice. Chapter 3 examines implementation of One Health practices that were presented in case studies of ongoing public health initiatives and research and interventions conducted in response to the COVID-19 pandemic. Chapter 4 explores current methods and challenges of integrating One Health ideology into existing epidemiological surveillance systems, as identified in two panel discussions. Chapter 5 summarizes two plenary presentations addressing potential steps to build the future One Health workforce and

---

[3] For more information, see https://www.who.int/ihr/procedures/joint-external-evaluations/en (accessed May 25, 2021).

experiential-learning initiatives currently under way. Chapter 6 summarizes four plenary presentations focusing on recently developed capabilities and innovation, collaboration, and investment efforts that could substantially mitigate future pandemic threats. Chapter 7 reviews the feasible goals and steps to improve future outbreak preparedness efforts that panelists discussed in breakout rooms.

Opening Remarks

One Health is a collaborative, multilevel, transdisciplinary approach to preventing, detecting, preparing for, and responding to outbreaks of infectious disease. Fundamentally, it recognizes the interconnectedness of the health of people, animals, plants, and their shared environment. One Health has the goal of achieving optimal health outcomes for people, animals, and the environment. It addresses diverse issues, including zoonotic diseases (those spread from animals to humans), emerging infectious diseases (e.g., coronavirus disease 2019 [COVID-19], antimicrobial resistance, food safety and food security, vector-borne diseases, wildlife diseases, and other shared health threats) (CDC, 2018). At the time of the workshop, the ongoing COVID-19 pandemic had raised worldwide awareness of the threat posed by infectious diseases and the need to improve prevention and response capacities. New opportunities have thus emerged to advance One Health initiatives and establish worldwide, collaborative pandemic prevention and response systems to enhance global health security.

Casey Barton Behravesh, director of the One Health office at the U.S. Centers for Disease Control and Prevention (CDC) and member of the workshop planning committee, gave welcoming remarks and explained that the workshop was organized with the goal of examining ways to systematize and integrate the One Health approach as part of the outbreak prevention, detection, preparedness, and response apparatus. This included examining successful implementations of One Health at local, national, and international levels; identifying gaps and challenges; and discussing future capacity building. Created in 1996, the Forum on Microbial Threats provides structured opportunities for discussion and scrutiny of critical—and possibly contentious—scientific and policy issues related to the prevention, detection, surveillance, and response to emerging and reemerging infectious diseases in people, plants, and animals, as well as the microbiome in health and disease. To this end, the Forum on Microbial Threats convenes workshops spanning a range of issues. Recent topics have included exploring the frontiers of innovation—including diagnostics, vaccines, and antimicrobials—to tackle microbial threats (NASEM, 2020); the growing understanding of how the interplay between people and microbes affects host physiology and noncommunicable diseases (NASEM, 2019a); and lessons learned from influenza pandemics and other major outbreaks that can be applied to better prepare countries for future pandemics (NASEM, 2019b).

Barton Behravesh provided context regarding the critical aspects of the One Health approach relevant to preparing for and responding to infectious disease outbreaks. She noted that even the fields of chronic disease, mental health, injury, occupational health, and noncommunicable diseases have benefited from a One Health approach. With applications at the local, regional, national, and global levels, One Health has gained momentum in every region across the world over the past decade, including within the United States.[4]

This momentum is in part driven by public health emergencies, such as Ebola virus disease and the COVID-19 pandemic, Barton Behravesh explained. Global health initiatives, such as the World Health Organization's (WHO's) International Health Regulations (WHO, 2008b) and the promotion of veterinary services performance by the World Organisation for Animal Health (OIE), have also increased awareness about the critical need for a One Health approach (OIE, 2012). Barton Behravesh noted that One Health is increasingly recognized by governments, the private sector, nongovernmental organizations, academic partners, and others as an effective way to combat health threats that affect people, animals, plants, and the shared environment. No single person, sector, or organization can adequately address issues at the human–animal–environment interface alone, Barton Behravesh maintained. Instead, effective preparedness and response efforts to these shared health threats require a One Health approach that emphasizes multi-sectoral collaboration and interdisciplinary partnerships. Collaboration, communication, and coordination across all relevant sectors and disciplines allow for effective planning and implementation of responses to zoonotic and infectious disease threats at all levels.

Emerging and endemic zoonotic diseases pose a threat to not only the health of people, animals, plants, and ecosystems but also global health security. Barton Behravesh explained that One Health is an important component of advancing the Global Health Security Agenda (GHSA),[5] a global effort to strengthen the world's ability to prevent, detect, and respond to infectious disease threats. Scientists estimate that 60 percent of known infectious diseases and 75 percent of emerging infectious diseases are zoonotic (Taylor et al., 2001). The COVID-19 pandemic has highlighted the value of One Health coordination, collaboration, and communication during a pandemic response, Barton Behravesh claimed. The impact of One

---

[4] For a review of challenges in the design and implementation of a One Health approach, see Ribeiro et al. (2019).

[5] For more information, see https://ghsagenda.org (accessed May 26, 2021).

Health collaboration can strengthen health systems, improve interagency communication and global health security, develop a proactive agenda, and maximize health outcomes for all.

Barton Behravesh also acknowledged that the transdisciplinary conservation medicine, EcoHealth, and planetary health approaches to protecting the health of humans, animals, plants, ecosystems, and the planet recognize that humans and animals share environmental challenges, the risk of infectious diseases, and other aspects of health. Hence, the EcoHealth, planetary health, and One Health initiatives are interrelated.

2

Keynote: One Health and Preventing Pandemics

Presented by Eric Goosby, University of California, San Francisco

The workshop featured a keynote address delivered during a session moderated by Casey Barton Behravesh. Eric Goosby, professor of medicine at the University of California, San Francisco, and former United Nations (UN) special envoy on tuberculosis (TB), provided an overview of the One Health concept and the shared responsibility across the international community that is needed to establish universal pandemic detection, response, and prevention capability. He outlined gaps in current surveillance and response efforts, described key sectors in creating a comprehensive system, and discussed the role of universal health coverage in such a system. Goosby also discussed strategies for increasing support of the One Health concept within the medical community, governments, and the general public. He cited examples pertaining to detecting and responding to the current coronavirus disease 2019 (COVID-19) pandemic throughout the presentation.

THE ONE HEALTH APPROACH

Goosby commented on the remarkable nature of the current moment, in which an orchestrated response to COVID-19 uses divergent strategies, funding lines, and human resources. Various geographic outbreaks are managed with a focus on outbreak intensity, while also addressing equity issues and compassionate service rollouts. The pandemic has required local, state, and national responses, as well as international efforts to understand how donor resources enter countries and match, synergize, or fail to fit with domestic resources. On a smaller scale, professionals are faced with determining how to integrate foundation and research efforts into creating strengthened local responses. A huge amount of surveillance, Goosby said, is required to understand what is taking place in the outbreak and response at any given time and geographical location. Applying that knowledge to decision making requires accessing and distributing substantial resources—including human, drug, and testing resources—at both state and city levels, a challenge that continues to present barriers. Goosby noted this was initially the case with testing supplies and currently is an issue with the vaccination effort.

The One Health approach can contribute to raising awareness of the need for an open and orchestrated understanding of how resources move and delivery systems interface with specific at-risk or target populations, said Goosby. Understanding how delivery systems interface—or fail to interface—with populations has been a challenge at the global level during outbreaks of human immunodeficiency virus (HIV), TB, and now COVID-19. In addition to strengthening the ability to detect outbreaks, effective surveillance efforts also inform a system that allows for expanding preparedness efforts and tailoring a response to the specific needs of the relevant populations. Goosby stated that this process is a recurring, repetitive challenge. The COVID-19 response capability has varied greatly in different parts of California, as was the case in most settings. Although prevention strategies often rely on the initial understanding of an issue, surveillance needs to continually inform decision makers and policy makers so they can institute corrective action in as close to real time as possible, said Goosby.

Approximately 60 percent of infectious diseases arise from pathogens shared with animals (Taylor et al., 2001). Goosby stated that, historically, paradigms for addressing zoonotic disease outbreaks—such as HIV, severe acute respiratory syndrome (SARS) and Middle East respiratory syndrome (MERS)—have largely been reactive. Current understanding of where a surveillance system is needed and would be most effective are limited because the mapping capacity required for this has not yet been developed. Furthermore, the ability to track how a potential threat changes over time is still largely aspirational, said Goosby, stating that economic losses resulting from outbreaks can be astounding—as highlighted by COVID-19. For comparison, the 2003 SARS outbreak that infected just over 8,000 people caused a global economic loss of $40–$54 billion (IOM, 2004). With the COVID-19 outbreak ongoing and economic impacts likely to persist for years, its total loss cannot yet be quantified. Goosby remarked that the economic effect on travel and entertainment alone, most notably in the airline industry, is catastrophic.

Goosby highlighted that antimicrobial resistance (AMR) is a topic for which One Health is applicable, since it has implications for both humans and animals. Animals in the United States consume two times the volume of medically important antibiotics that humans do (O'Neill, 2016). On the human side, AMR is particularly relevant in the context of TB, for which the annual rate of AMR-attributable deaths is projected to be as high as 10 million by 2050 (Spellberg et al., 2013). Given evolving understandings about AMR's relevance to both the animal industry and human health, Goosby suggested that an integrated approach to AMR data in policy decisions could be useful. Furthermore, consensus is needed on current readiness to implement surveillance capability through the International Health Regulations (IHR). He added that increased transparency would enhance the ability to monitor outbreaks in countries lacking continuously running surveillance systems that uniformly cover the geography (Review on Antimicrobial Resistance, 2015; Solomon and Oliver, 2014; WHO, 2014).

Nonprofit organizations are largely responsible for raising awareness of outbreaks in the locations in which they operate, said Goosby. Much discussion has centered on this dynamic since the Ebola challenges of 2014–2016.[1] However, this has not resulted in a pivot toward an effective, sustainable surveillance system, despite the 2005 IHR describing it, Goosby noted (WHO, 2008a). Typically, a virus is not detected at the point when it jumps from an animal reservoir to a human host but rather when an infected individual engages the medical delivery system. This detection can occur long after the virus has had the opportunity to embed and spread within a human population, so resources should be mobilized to enable the surveillance system to operate rapidly in front of a pathogen as it begins to move into humans, he added.

ONE HEALTH PANDEMIC RESPONSE FRAMEWORK

The ethos of the One Health approach is to provide detection, response, and prevention capabilities at the global, national, and local levels, said Goosby. This involves orchestration that is multi-sectoral, transdisciplinary, and collaborative. Transparency and accountability are essential to building system integrity. He noted that it is important to be able to reveal weaknesses and vulnerabilities without criticism or ridicule, instead meeting these with an attempt to better understand and strengthen the response. Given the disparities and inequitable distribution of capabilities throughout the globe, shared responsibility across the international community is the only realistic method of creating a system of preparedness and alerts for emerging threats, said Goosby. He contended that the assumption that individual sovereign nations can be independently responsible for the entire

---

[1] The 2014–2016 Ebola epidemic in West Africa caused more than 11,300 deaths in Guinea, Liberia, and Sierra Leone. More information about this outbreak can be found at https://www.cdc.gov/media/releases/2016/p0707-history-ebola-response.html (accessed March 26, 2021).

complement from outbreak detection to response—without regional or global support—leads to less successful efforts, as multiple examples in the attempt to mount various regional COVID-19 responses have indicated.

Improving Pandemic Detection

Given that a majority of human infectious diseases arise from pathogens shared with wild or domestic animals (Taylor et al., 2001), Goosby pointed out that the risk of disease emergence exists virtually everywhere, not just in low-income countries. A global surveillance system would be able to detect pathogens before they reach domesticated animals—where they have the opportunity to spread to humans. He said he understands that the World Health Organization (WHO) and the UN are discussing the ability to fund and support the level of global orchestration that such surveillance requires. In the United States, the Biden administration is working to convene a specific discussion about threat detection and response from a regional perspective. Goosby added that this is the first time in his career that high-level talks about pathogen detection efforts are taking place, and he was eager to see these pivot into a funded, sustained priority.[2]

Global Actions in Pandemic Detection

Goosby emphasized that improving pandemic detection demands new global action. The COVID-19 pandemic has revealed the frailty of existing global detection mechanisms. IHR systems were weak due to governments lacking motivation to share public health risks, Goosby noted, and post-COVID-19 efforts can improve upon this by incentivizing the sharing of outbreak data. WHO should reinvigorate IHR—placing greater focus on intersectional equity—and the UN should establish health security infrastructure, said Goosby.[3] These steps would create surveillance systems capable of discerning an outbreak, notifying authorities, quantifying the concern, and prompting action from WHO. This would include an announcement, evaluation, and reconsideration of whether the threat does indeed reach emergency level. In an established emergency, resources would be released to converge on the site to enable continuous surveillance that would feed and inform an international understanding of the threat.

---

[2] A recent report of the G20 High Level Independent Panel on Financing the Global Commons for Pandemic Preparedness and Response (published after the workshop, in June 2021) addresses the issue of permanent funding for global disease surveillance directly. The report, "A Global Deal for our Pandemic Age," can be found at https://pandemic-financing.org/report/foreword (accessed August 9, 2021).

[3] The definition of intersectionality as it applies to public health can be found at http://www.ncchpp.ca/docs/2015_Ineg_Ineq_Intersectionnalite_En.pdf (accessed July 7, 2021).

Goosby noted that rather than duplicating capability in multiple areas, regions require the ability to move resources to the problem, allowing for rapidly expanding capabilities in the source country.

Regional talent should be pre-identified and prepared to respond to an alarm within hours—assessing, reporting, and initiating an infusion of additional resources to better define and respond to findings, said Goosby. This must be a shared responsibility, which requires a high degree of commitment, Goosby asserted. To date, relying on individual sovereign nations to establish the full continuum of services and capability for surveillance has largely been unsuccessful. Discussions are taking place on incentivizing surveillance, including generating definitions of the specific incentives. The impact of surveillance on health security is often influential in driving developed countries to generate resources for the global detection effort, because governments and appropriators are generally more willing to contribute funding when it is contextualized in terms of security. He noted that many medical professionals view security considerations as outside their comfort zone. However, as public health and medical considerations may not come into play for security decision-making groups, Goosby suggested that medical professionals include security considerations in their discussions. Goosby added that security-focused and public health–focused thinking can enhance one another, but since these are distinct communities, attention should be given to the processes needed to move toward synergy.

Local Actions in Pandemic Detection

The necessary increase in detection capability will need to evolve locally, said Goosby. Monitoring all humans, animals, and environments on a global level would likely be unfeasible, so greater sophistication is required to address various surveillance challenges—for example, strengthening the capacity for earlier detection and developing an alarm system that generates regional alerts to trigger capacity support on a global level. New approaches and novel technology could empower local communities and support traditional surveillance capabilities, especially in hot spots (Allen et al., 2017). Examining COVID-19 trends in big data has enabled greater understanding of the movement and purchasing patterns of people within a given geography in California, leading to predictions of infection and hospitalization surges. The capacity to predict the impact of increased population accumulation—such as during the Christmas holidays—on hospital delivery systems has now become quite accurate. Technology such as tracking the purchasing patterns on cell phones will add another lens to the ability to be more specific in anticipating threats, he added.

Strengthening Pandemic Response

Goosby stated that many countries, including the United States, have limited contact tracing capabilities, as has been evident during outbreaks of COVID-19 and TB (Hale et al., 2021), and some countries have none. Limited contact tracing impedes the ability to limit new infections. Prior to COVID-19, nearly 40 percent of large emerging disease events were linked to lack of public health infrastructure (Bogich et al., 2012). To avoid similar failures in future pandemics, countries should strengthen their health systems to enable a rapid and coherent response, said Goosby. He noted that in California's Bay Area, high COVID-19 infection rates have hampered contact tracing efforts, which are less effective during large surges of infections. He anticipated that the decreasing infection rate will reinvigorate the utility of contact tracing. In California, this case-finding contact strategy was planned to begin with six counties before moving to a regional level, with surveillance informing each stage of lifting containment measures. Goosby pointed out that this is a shift from the last three infection surges in California, where surveillance did not inform reopening plans. This pattern exemplifies the shared responsibility of a regional response, which should be modeled and implemented at the global level, he added.

Key Response Sectors

Several sectors have key roles in response efforts through continuous and episodic engagement. National governments, which remain the entities responsible for responding to outbreaks, have a line of accountability that can be invoked. Goosby noted that governments are responsible for the population in a way that other sectors are not; thus, they should be accountable for initiating and leading health responses. He continued that local, state, provincial, and national governments are critical partners in orchestrating procurement and distribution systems at scale. Academia can engage schools of medicine, public health, and veterinary medicine to lower barriers in applying the best science, data solutions, policies, and technologies for in-country implementation. Additionally, academia offers specific skill sets needed to collect, aggregate, and analyze data. This analysis can create feedback loops with policy makers, identifying mistakes in implementation and recommending improvements, thus creating self-correcting systems. Goosby emphasized that such partnerships are needed between government and local academia to establish sustainable patterns. He added that all the countries he has worked in have had pockets of capability that should be recognized, expanded, and leveraged, such as those that have driven progress in the past 30 years in responding to HIV and TB epidemics. Pivoting to finding regional talent—as opposed to bringing in an academic medical center from thousands of miles away—can help to evolve and mature the delivery of care, said Goosby.

The nonprofit sector also plays a role in establishing credibility in recommended services. Local community-based organizations are able to access populations that historically have been difficult to identify and retain for care over time, making these organizations valuable partners in response efforts. The private sector can harness the strengths and networks of business, investors, and enterprise to address identified health priorities in partnership with government. However, Goosby noted that public–private partnerships can be relied on too heavily, and—given that the private sector rarely holds a mandate to sustain a response—it can be difficult for the government to hold the private sector accountable. Thus, while the private sector can bolster response efforts by providing financial resources and capacity for procurement and distribution, Goosby said the appropriateness of roles should be considered in establishing such partnerships.

The health diplomacy and advocacy sector can contribute to engaging constructively with ministries of health and other parties to identify health priorities, critical implementation issues, and barriers to success. Goosby remarked that it can elevate the role of global health awareness in diplomatic discourse between countries. In the United States, work is under way to understand how to use a health diplomacy platform more effectively to discuss expanding national-level capabilities in determining international-level programming priorities. Many European countries also consider this an area that needs to be leveraged more aggressively, said Goosby.

Universal Health Care Coverage and Pandemic Prevention

The prevention element of pandemic preparedness is difficult to anticipate, Goosby noted. The surveillance system is critical in enabling the ability to mount a counter-response. Discussions of pandemic prevention inevitably lead to the role of community health workers and primary care in supporting local surveillance efforts and containment strategies. While it is logical to contend with one disease via specific health disciplines that may be excellent, though siloed, Goosby maintained that prevention efforts cannot stop there. An integrated, sustainable portfolio of services is beneficial, as many individuals with infectious diseases, such as HIV, TB, or COVID-19, also have other diseases and comorbidities. Clinics that perform disease-specific services require people with multiple health issues to move from one site to another to receive care for their different conditions and needs (e.g., family planning, HIV, TB, hypertension, diabetes, coronary artery disease). However, most programs focusing on a single disease have not yet matured to meet the full spectrum of needs. The universal health coverage (UHC) movement, the One Health concept, and the global health community at large are converging upon the recognition—underscored by the COVID-19 pandemic—that finding ways to meet the diverse needs of people who are already in existing care delivery systems, while also being positioned to expand in response to new threats, represents a major challenge. UHC ensures accessible, equitable, affordable care, particularly for specific underserved communities, and enables coordination of programs and stakeholders, said Goosby. Therefore, UHC is a critical component of pandemic prevention (Binagwaho and Mathewos, 2020).

GLOBAL INTERCONNECTEDNESS

The COVID-19 pandemic, like any global crisis, serves as a reminder that the problems of some humans are the problems of all humans, said Goosby (Reid et al., 2021). In a globalized world, no one country alone can effectively respond to human, animal, plant, and ecosystem health threats. To prevent and respond to future pandemic threats, Goosby surmised, coordinated, multi-sectoral strategies are needed that are inclusive, participatory, and based on principles of shared responsibility. For most countries, acting alone to achieve needed actions is not realistic, which speaks to the role WHO and the UN play in orchestrating the identification of unmet needs and invoking shared responsibilities to fill those needs as a global community. This includes the shared global responsibility to understand morbidity, inequities, disparities, and impact as an outbreak moves through the population. Efficiency in understanding and communicating morbidity and inequities establishes credibility with populations, even more so when differences in outbreak dynamics are reflected in allocation decisions. Establishing these connections is challenging, he added, especially on the international scale. A conduit is needed that can present, solidify, and document data regarding needs while simultaneously creating a line of accountability. Goosby said that he anticipates that the One Health platform will become increasingly important in this effort.

DISCUSSION

Student Engagement

Barton Behravesh asked Goosby how he might approach engaging students in One Health. He replied that, from his position at an academic medical center, he recognizes that medical students, residents, and fellows are the future of One Health, and thus efforts to promote this global thinking among students could help the platform gain traction. While students may intuitively recognize the need for this pivot, introducing these ideas during medical rounds can socialize this type of thinking. Goosby noted he believes the current period is one of bridging medical cultures and perspectives to create synergies. He added that academic medical centers need to open their divisions and acknowledge the role that research institutes and centers can play in augmenting more traditional departments of medicine. Based on his conversations, Goosby said, many deans and chancellors also see this as a necessary step moving forward.

Building Consensus for a Global Health System

A participant asked about the extent to which disparity of opinion regarding the global health system harms One Health efforts. Goosby responded that discussion of resource expansion is difficult because government budgets are already strained. Adding new priorities requires reorganizing current priorities. However, Goosby noted how helping governments to understand how One Health dovetails with security may help to shift discussion of government appropriations and increase willingness to acknowledge the existing resource deficit when looking at both areas simultaneously. For professionals who are not considering issues of health, the security component can catalyze new understandings of health threats. He encouraged medical professionals to develop an understanding of security language and threat perception, as synergy in those areas can lead to funding for an essential new system.

Tracking Movement and Purchasing Patterns

Another participant asked Goosby to elaborate on how cell phones, movement, and purchasing patterns can be used for detection and surveillance and what implementation would look like. Goosby noted that in San Francisco, purchases taking place after Thanksgiving were tracked. This information was not specific to individuals but instead was used to evaluate overall buying patterns, such as from online retailers or in stores. Such patterns reflect how much interaction people are having. As interaction increased, the number of new infections likewise increased within 2–3 weeks. Goosby stated that at the local level, patterns of increased interaction were used as a surrogate marker of increased spread, indicating the need to prepare for a surge. Similarly, cell phone location patterns can provide data to estimate infection rates, which can be added to the compilation of information used for decisions about, for example, lifting restrictions as well as evaluating public compliance with restrictions and determining the appropriate timing for lifting restrictions. He added that surveillance on face mask use has been conducted via images on closed circuit televisions.

Influencing the International Animal Trade

Given that many vertebrate species are traded internationally, a participant asked how to prevent the spread of infectious diseases without negatively impacting a trade that is central to cultural traditions, livelihoods, and economic activities around the world. Goosby replied that understanding and delivering pertinent science to decision makers and the populations holding such cultural beliefs should be conducted transparently, aggressively, and continuously. Targeting local leaders to be part of the process means that they can become spokespeople for connecting the risk of infection with certain practices. An iterative, community-oriented approach can be useful because governments do not naturally gravitate to these types of efforts; however, HIV outbreaks have demonstrated the value of initiating dialogue with communities to identify and retain patients, which can reduce the number of deaths over time. He added that when faced with difficult outcomes, people will eventually become convinced that changes are needed if the potential consequences are brought to their attention. Encouraging ministries of health and governments to perform this type of surveillance can move the agenda forward, he added. However, the overwhelming majority of current global health data efforts involve collecting and aggregating data that are never actually analyzed.

Increasing Public Awareness of One Health

Barton Behravesh asked how to bring the concept of One Health to the awareness of the general public. Goosby noted that efforts such as *The Lancet*'s One Health Commission have been helpful in bringing literature to specific, targeted communities (Amuasi et al., 2020a). Regarding a strategy for reaching the general population, the interconnected systems of the planet should be presented more comprehensively. For instance, the educational system is segmented and stratified, while the interconnectedness of the planet is a theme that should be reflected in every discipline. Professionals who develop curricula can find ways to relate it to areas of study ranging from science to social studies to literature. Noting the use of a Muppet character who has HIV on the U.S. children's television series *Sesame Street*, Goosby said that educating the general public about health can begin in early childhood.[4] Communications professionals can use media to socialize concepts for general audiences. He remarked that institutions could increase visibility of this topic by hiring advertising firms skilled in making messages memorable, but few efforts are currently under way to increase general awareness.

---

[4] More information about HIV education on *Sesame Street* can be found at https://www.unicef.org/media/media_16631.html (accessed March 28, 2021).

Encouraging Sharing of Outbreak Data

A participant asked about efforts to incentivize sharing outbreak data on a global scale during pandemics. Goosby noted that this is a new topic for discussion, with few if any efforts yet under way. Countries that are competing at every level for resources to address legitimate unmet needs should be a part of the process of determining country-specific incentives, he added, and nations that cannot afford the investment will need assistance. This process should be conducted with—not for—countries to establish national-level ownership. Barton Behravesh asked how the United States can leverage its global leadership role to encourage open and honest disclosure of outbreaks in other countries. Goosby replied that WHO, the UN, and some foundations are in a position to influence reaction to outbreaks. Currently, a punitive blame reflex remains, as evidenced in the reaction to COVID-19, in which political blame-placing began almost immediately, Goosby lamented. He believed that this reaction undermined efforts to analyze whether opportunities had existed to identify the outbreak earlier, to the detriment of understanding where alert systems were effective or inadequate.

Goosby said that to progress toward a comprehensive surveillance system, surveillance gaps should be aggressively mapped. If WHO is empowered to take on this effort, it will require assistance from major donors; such efforts should focus on understanding how new threats move through the population, whether these could reach the global population, and how to contain them. Blaming is counterproductive to these efforts, he added. Sufficient transparency is needed to be able to detect and alert the world of threats early enough to contain them. This transparency relies on building trust among countries that they will not be criticized or punished for revealing their vulnerabilities. This type of shift is achievable given the political will to do so, he said.

Current Status of One Health Implementation

Barton Behravesh remarked that the One Health movement has been ongoing for almost 20 years, but implementation remains a major challenge. The features that are fundamental to operationalizing One Health (i.e., multifactorial, collaborative, transdisciplinary, accountable, and shared responsibility) can be difficult for middle- and low-income countries to establish, because they require commitment from diverse sectors. She asked about examples of locations where progress is being made. Additionally, she queried which challenges are the greatest in broad, proactive implementation of One Health. Goosby responded that the greatest challenge to achieving an acceptable response is countries' unwillingness to expand their capabilities. This specifically relates to governments and the ministries of health—which are at the core of the response—and civil society, which can implement steps toward One Health and teach others to do so. Building capability should involve engaging these sectors from the start, said Goosby. He highlighted Rwanda as an example of a country that has established self-determination in these efforts. Rather than allowing multinational nongovernmental organizations to implement programs, Rwanda created its own platforms for addressing HIV and TB outbreaks and used these as a foundation for a COVID-19 response. Goosby stated that Rwanda takes the role of "doer," which positions it ahead of other nations in the region in effectively responding to outbreaks.

3

One Health in Praxis

The second session of the workshop examined three case studies of the implementation of One Health practices, integration into public health systems, and strategies for mitigating relevant barriers. Dana Wiltz-Beckham, director of the Office of Science, Surveillance, and Technology at Harris County Public Health (HCPH), Texas, United States, described the One Health initiative at her organization. She provided an overview of its structure, growth, and responses to various outbreaks and natural disasters in recent years. Supaporn Wacharapluesadee, researcher at Thai Red Cross Emerging Infectious Diseases Health Science Centre (TRC-EID), King Chulalongkorn Memorial Hospital, Bangkok, Thailand, outlined the roles of discovery, diagnosis, and research and development in early detection and control of an outbreak. She discussed the expansion of testing capacity in Thailand and reviewed research findings on coronaviruses in bats and pangolins. Thierry Nyatanyi, senior advisor of the Africa Task Force for Novel Coronavirus at the Africa Centres for Disease Control and Prevention (Africa CDC), outlined Rwanda's coordinated response to coronavirus disease 2019 (COVID-19). He discussed numerous measures, such as a rapid scale-up of epidemiological surveillance—including severe acute respiratory syndrome coronavirus 2 (SARS-CoV-2) testing—and outlined strategies for future improvements in health system resilience. The panel was moderated by Kent Kester, vice president and head of translational science and biomarkers at Sanofi Pasteur.

OPERATIONALIZING ONE HEALTH AT A LOCAL LEVEL

Presented by Dana Wiltz-Beckham, HCPH (Texas, United States)

Wiltz-Beckham described the population, infrastructure, and weather patterns of Harris County, Texas. She outlined the organizational structure of HCPH and detailed the offices and divisions that participate in its One Health initiative. Providing examples of HCPH responses to zoonotic outbreaks and natural disasters, she described the implementation of the One Health model and contrasted this collaborative approach with the siloed approach it had previously used.

Features of Harris County, Texas

Located in southeast Texas near the Gulf of Mexico, Harris County spans more than 1,700 square miles and contains 4.7 million people. Wiltz-Beckham described Harris County as one of the most diverse communities in the United States, with more than 145 languages spoken among its residents. Houston, the fourth-largest city in the United States, is located in Harris County and has two large public health agencies: Houston Health Department and HCPH.[1] Houston is also home to Texas Medical Center, the largest medical center in the world, in addition to one of the world's largest seaports, two international airports, and the nation's largest concentration of petrochemical facilities. HCPH houses the largest refugee health screening program in Texas. Wiltz-Beckham noted that these details paint a picture of the diverse and complex nature of Harris County. Due to its proximity to the Gulf of Mexico, Harris County is the "gateway of hurricanes," said Wiltz-Beckham. In addition to hurricane impacts, the county has been affected by incidents related to its petrochemical facilities. Over the past 4 years, the area has experienced several crises, with impacts currently ongoing: Hurricane Harvey in 2017, a petrochemical fire in 2019, COVID-19, and Winter Storm Uri in 2021.

HCPH Organizational Structure

HCPH comprises five divisions specific to subject matter. The Disease Control and Clinical Prevention (DCCP) Division includes the tuberculosis and refugee health programs. The Environmental Public Health (EPH) Division conducts sanitation and inspection services. The other divisions are Nutrition and Chronic Disease Prevention, Veterinary Public Health (VPH),

---

[1] More information about Harris County Public Health can be found at https://publichealth.harriscountytx.gov (accessed March 29, 2021).

and the Mosquito and Vector Control Division (MVCD). Additionally, HCPH has five offices that transect across divisions: Communications, Education and Engagement; Finance Services and Support; Policy and Planning; Public Health Preparedness and Response; and the Office of Science Surveillance and Technology. Wiltz-Beckham noted that HCPH is a comprehensive local health department, offering a full range of services, including veterinary public services, animal control, preparedness, outreach, dental, HIV prevention, mosquito vector control, inspection of pools and nuisance complaints, sanitarian services, and immunizations.

Wiltz-Beckham outlined the offices and divisions that contribute to the One Health initiative at HCPH. The Office of Science Surveillance and Technology addresses epidemiology, tracking and monitoring, and data housing, and also serves as a repository for science-related items. Disease Control and Clinical Prevention provides physician services, and Nutrition and Chronic Disease Prevention offers mental health expertise. VPH provides animal control services and responds to safety codes related to rabies. MVCD works to decrease disease spread at the source. EPH ensures food safety, offers lead poisoning prevention efforts, and works to increase the safety and health equity of the built environment.

One Health Responses at HCPH

Discussions around One Health began at HCPH in 2013, and operationalization was initiated in 2014, said Wiltz-Beckham. With more than 60 percent of infectious diseases in the United States resulting from animals, HCPH routinely addresses zoonotic diseases (Taylor et al., 2001).

West Nile Virus Response

Wiltz-Beckham noted that before adopting the One Health approach, HCPH staff worked in silos (see Figure 3-1). For example, if the epidemiology department's surveillance program or epidemiology (EPI) team received a positive lab result for West Nile virus, the program would confirm the case and proceed to investigate it, educate the infected individual, contact the hospital, run EPI processes, and report the case to the state health department; in turn, the state health department would report it to the U.S. Centers for Disease Control and Prevention (CDC). Independent of those processes, Wiltz-Beckham explained, MVCD tested mosquitoes for West Nile virus and sprayed accordingly, while sanitarians (officials responsible for public health) and animal control officers out on routine calls may have observed old tires—known breeding grounds for mosquitoes. Each office or division would conduct these activities independently, without communicating. She described the implementation of the One Health initiative as

Before One Health

 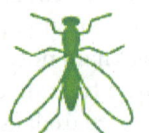 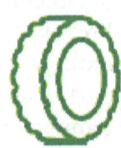

A person's positive test result for West Nile Virus arrives at the health department | Mosquitos at the health department's entomology lab test positive | Old tires are observed by a department animal control officer while on a routine call

After One Health

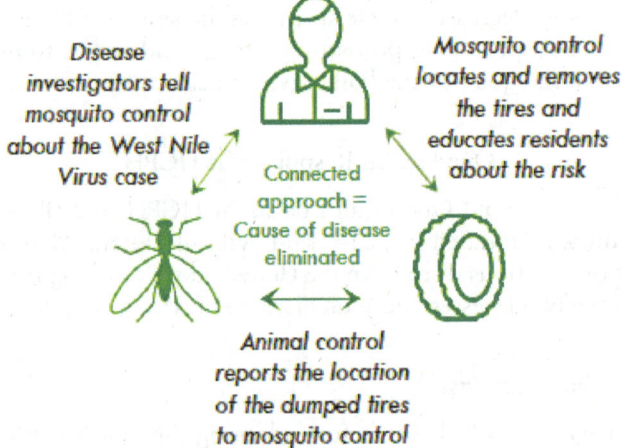

FIGURE 3-1 Harris County Public Health Department's response to West Nile virus: Before and after the One Health approach.
SOURCE: Wiltz-Beckham presentation, February 23, 2021.

breaking down these silos through collaboration. Now, when surveillance and the EPI team identify a positive case of West Nile virus, they notify MVCD. Wiltz-Beckham noted that a lack of data sharing by zip code, which designates location in the United States, has historically been a barrier to effective response efforts at HCPH and also at the local, state, and federal levels. Upon notification, MVCD can investigate the location of the positive case and determine whether spraying is required. Animal control officers and sanitarians now report sightings of old tires to MVCD, who remove the tires or treat the area with mosquito dunks to prevent breeding.

Zika Virus Response

The response to the 2016 outbreak of Zika virus is another example of the collaboration One Health has brought to HCPH, said Wiltz-Beckham. The department formed a multidisciplinary team that included law enforcement, policy staff, VPH, the EPI team, EPH, and medical professionals. The team trained and worked together to develop a Zika response. Partnering with home associations and places of worship, the communication and education outreach team went into neighborhoods to hold health fairs and teach residents how mosquitoes breed. Responding to this public health issue with focus on equity, she explained, areas were analyzed with an index of social vulnerability, and locations with high scores were targeted for testing mosquitoes. When positive cases were identified, the team studied the relevant areas. The response shifted from low-tech (such as outreach and education) to high-tech strategies. These included partnering with Microsoft to develop a system that captures mosquitoes, determines sex, and measures wing movement to identify species—as various species carry different viruses.

Rabies Response

Wiltz-Beckham noted that the United States has effectively decreased rabies cases over time, but rabies still persists. In Harris County, the majority of cases occur in bats, she said, with 7–10 percent of bats submitted each year for rabies testing carrying the virus. Once an animal tests positive, a multidisciplinary team is alerted, and animal control officers go to the area to conduct outreach services. For example, HCPH physicians communicate with veterinarians in an effort to ensure that anyone who came into contact with the rabid bat is evaluated. In cases where rabies post-exposure treatment is needed, the physicians assist those individuals in accessing required treatment. Wildlife experts, community outreach, and the media also have roles in the response.

Hurricane Harvey Response

More than 3 years after the 2017 disaster, Wiltz-Beckham said Harris County continues its recovery efforts in response to Hurricane Harvey. Involving multi-agency coordination, HCPH has collaborated with organizations throughout the country and the nation. Community-engagement efforts include an HCPH mobile health village that provides a "one-stop shop" of public health outreach services, including rabies vaccinations and microchipping for dogs; dental evaluations for children; flu shots; registration for social benefits, such as the Special Supplemental Nutrition Program for Women, Infants, and Children; and information on preparedness. After Hurricane Harvey, the mobile health village was set up throughout Harris County. Additionally, HCPH conducted surveillance in shelters for people and pets displaced by the hurricane. Mosquito control, environmental health, and animal management services have also been part of HCPH's Hurricane Harvey response.

COVID-19 Response

Wiltz-Beckham stated that HCPH's response to the COVID-19 pandemic began on January 9, 2020, and has been continually updated since. The surveillance and EPI team grew from 25 staff members to nearly 500. The social services department works with individuals who need to be quarantined or isolated but do not have spaces in which to do so. Pet owners are educated regarding the risks of COVID-19 to animals. They also offer testing and vaccination services and, with a specific focus on ensuring equity, addressing underserved areas lacking these services, she added. The Office of Policy and Planning develops policy guidance and works with Communication and Engagement to release timely information to the public via news media and social media. The Health Alert Network provides dental, veterinary, and health care education information. A seroprevalence project is currently studying humans with COVID-19 antibodies, while another pilot project is under way to investigate prevalence and seroprevalence in animals. Lastly, HCPH is learning from best practices shared by China and South Korea.

Winter Storm Uri Response

Texas was recovering from Winter Storm Uri, which severely affected the state in February 2021. The surveillance and EPI team monitored warming centers (short-term emergency shelters that operate during inclement weather events) for viruses. Wiltz-Beckham noted that HCPH provided services to the homeless population and to animals during the storm, as well as offering mental health services. Carbon monoxide poisoning was also addressed.

One Health Growth at HCPH

For the past 14 years, HCPH has hosted an annual conference. What began as a small workshop at the local zoo grew into a large veterinary conference; in 2017, it evolved to its current iteration as a One Health conference, bringing together professionals from veterinary, medical, environmental, and public health disciplines.[2] The most recent conference was held in October 2020 (virtually, due to the pandemic). Wiltz-Beckham noted overwhelmingly positive feedback from participants regarding sessions on emerging pathogens and microbial threats.

Wiltz-Beckham stated that HCPH is implementing various One Health initiatives at the local level. The organization began without any designated One Health staff positions, added part-time coordination assistance, and now has full-time One Health and global health coordinators. As future pathogens emerge, additional work will be needed to address these and increases in cases and risk, she said. For example, in the United States, disease cases from infected mosquitoes, ticks, and fleas tripled from 2004 to 2016 (Rosenberg et al., 2018). Meeting such challenges will require increased funding, vector control, research, and education. Advocating for the continued growth of One Health, HCPH is working toward establishing proactive policies and funding support that is flexible and appropriate to build necessary capacity at the local level. This involves educating the governing body about One Health's role and importance. Wiltz-Beckham added that HCPH continues to hold multidisciplinary conversations and improve response evaluation to identify gaps and potential solutions.

MULTI-SECTORAL ENGAGEMENT IN THE COVID-19 OUTBREAK RESPONSE IN THAILAND

Presented by Supaporn Wacharapluesadee, King Chulalongkorn Memorial Hospital (Bangkok, Thailand)

Wacharapluesadee discussed components of outbreak detection and control. She outlined efforts to expand surveillance and testing in Thailand, highlighting additional capacity-building measures that have taken place since the pandemic began. Reviewing research of coronaviruses in bats and pangolins, she also detailed findings linking the virus to bats.

The "Three Ds" of Outbreak Detection and Control

Wacharapluesadee outlined the "three Ds" of early detection and control of an outbreak—discovery, diagnosis, and research and development—and described how Thailand effectively performed these in its COVID-19

---

[2] More information about HCPH's One Health Conference can be found at https://publichealth.harriscountytx.gov/Services-Programs/All-Programs/One-Health-Conference (accessed March 29, 2021).

response. *Discovery* involves Thailand's early detection efforts, which are provided by a partnership of the Department of Disease Control (DDC), the Department of Medical Science (DMSc), and TRC-EID, which is located at King Chulalongkorn Memorial Hospital and Chulalongkorn University. *Diagnosis* pertains to outbreak control. Wacharapluesadee explained that reference laboratories in the diagnostic laboratory network, including DMSc, TRC-EID, and universities, expanded rapidly to include provincial public health laboratories and private laboratories to deliver 24-hour turnaround time. She said that this enabled DDC to respond promptly by investigating contact cases, resulting in better control and containment. *Research and development* provide knowledge to strengthen early detection efforts that eventually lead to diagnosis and also inform response efforts. During the pandemic, the U.S. Agency for International Development (USAID) and the U.S. Defense Threat Reduction Agency contributed funding to expand Thailand's capacity to cope with the emerging infectious diseases, Wacharapluesadee noted. Additionally, a national, multi-sectoral collaboration among the Ministry of Public Health, private hospitals, and the academic research center expanded surveillance of variants of SARS-CoV-2 that cause COVID-19.

The PREDICT Diagnostic Approach

Spanning from 2010 to 2019, USAID's PREDICT research project was implemented in 35 countries at high risk for zoonotic disease emergence, including Thailand, said Wacharapluesadee.[3] In April 2020, it was extended to provide emergency support to Thailand during the COVID-19 pandemic. Aiming to improve surveillance by strengthening capacity for sampling and laboratory detection of known viruses, PREDICT-Thailand efforts resulted in 59 staff members trained in One Health skills, 678 humans and 3,288 animals sampled, 42,610 tests administered, and 448 viruses detected (mostly coronaviruses, both novel and previously identified). To detect viruses, Wacharapluesadee explained, the PREDICT diagnostic approach used a family-wide polymerase chain reaction (PCR) using a consensus primer, which provided broad amplification of multiple genetically related pathogens, including previously unidentified ones—enabling both known and novel viruses to be detected within the same PCR reaction.

Wacharapluesadee presented a table of surveillance results in wildlife she and her team tested over 5 years for several virus families, including coronaviruses, filoviruses, flaviviruses, influenza viruses, and paramyxoviruses

---

[3] More information about PREDICT can be found at https://www.usaid.gov/sites/default/files/documents/1864/predict-global-flyer-508.pdf and https://ohi.vetmed.ucdavis.edu/programs-projects/predict-project (both accessed March 30, 2021).

(PREDICT Consortium, 2020, p. 540). A heat map of the findings indicated that the majority of positive samples for coronaviruses were found in bats, she said. This process taught her and her team how to detect novel coronaviruses in bats, which would inform procedures for humans. The coronavirus family-wide PCR was used to discover the Middle East respiratory syndrome (MERS) coronavirus in 2012, she added (Zaki et al., 2012).

Discovery of the COVID-19 Virus

Learnings from the MERS discovery, coupled with her findings about coronaviruses in bats, Wacharapluesadee said she was able to perform family-wide PCR detection on an unknown virus that the Thai government asked her laboratory to identify in January 2020. The workflow involved the collaboration of three national laboratories. DDC's Bamrasnaradura Infectious Diseases Institute was responsible for detecting all known respiratory pathogens from the same sample. Two other samples were sent to Wacharapluesadee's laboratory at TRC-EID, where she performed family-wide PCR for coronavirus and influenza virus and next-generation sequencing.[4] The DMSc also tested for unknown pneumonia. She explained that when a pathogen is unknown, different detection protocols are used. The discovery of the first COVID-19 case in Thailand began on January 8, 2020, she said, when specimens tested with viral family PCR assays were positive for a coronavirus. The following day, Wacharapluesadee stated, sequence matching with the gene bank indicated that the virus shared 83–90 percent identity with coronaviruses found in bats. It did not match any human viruses, she explained, and at that point, the coronavirus sequence from Wuhan, China, was not yet available. On January 11, 2020, China shared the data of the virus that caused the unknown pneumonia in Wuhan; her laboratory then reanalyzed the sample and found it was a 100 percent match with that disease. The next day, TRC-EID and DMSc performed next-generation whole genome sequence analysis, with both laboratories confirming that the virus was the same as that found in Wuhan.

Thailand's COVID-19 Detection Capacity

Wacharapluesadee stated that with Thailand's diagnostic network expanding to include more than 200 laboratories in 76 provinces,

---

[4] "Next-generation sequencing," or "high-throughput sequencing," is an umbrella term used to refer to modern nucleic acid sequencing techniques (distinct from the traditional Sanger sequencing method). For more information, see https://www.ebi.ac.uk/training/online/courses/functional-genomics-ii-common-technologies-and-data-analysis-methods/next-generation-sequencing (accessed July 7, 2021).

COVID-19 PCR results can be delivered within 24 hours. She noted that an enhanced biosafety level 2 molecular laboratory has been created in the past year to perform COVID-19 testing. Thailand's laboratory network is able to target multiple genes and perform high-throughput real-time PCR. The nation's capability to perform rapid, quality-controlled testing enables effective outbreak control efforts. Led by Thailand's national laboratory, a multi-sectoral collaboration is conducting surveillance for SARS-CoV-2 variants. Wacharapluesadee presented a table of surveillance findings generated by a partnership between TRC-EID, DDC, and private hospitals working to identify variants entering the country via the airport. Targeting people who are quarantined by the state after traveling abroad, the collaboration is able to report detected variations within 5 days of arrival at the airport, she said.

Bat and Pangolin Coronavirus Research

The horseshoe bat, *Rhinolophus affinis*, was thought to be a probable origin of SARS-CoV-2 (Zhou et al., 2020). Found in south China, Thailand, Cambodia, and Indonesia, this bat can become infected with RaTG13—a betacoronavirus that shows 96 percent nucleotide identity to SARS-CoV-2 found in humans (Ge et al., 2016). To fight viruses related to SARS-CoV-2 in Thailand, Wacharapluesadee and her team have been working to identify the origin of virus variants. The Department of National Parks, Wildlife, and Plant Conservation, Chulalongkorn University, and Kasetsart University began an international collaboration with Duke-National University of Singapore's Emerging Infectious Diseases Program in June 2020 to study bats in connection with SARS-CoV-2 (Wacharapluesadee et al., 2021). Wacharapluesadee and a team of researchers went to east Thailand, where they collected 100 *Rhinolophus acuminatus*, or acuminate horseshoe bats, from a cave. The team took blood samples for serology surveillance and rectal swabs for PCR and genetic study; 13 of the 100 bats tested positive for coronaviruses. She continued by stating that researchers sequenced the 290-base pair RdRp gene and identified a close relationship to both the human SARS-CoV-2 and the RaTG13 found in bats—with homologies of 95.9 percent and 96.2 percent, respectively. When whole-genome sequencing was performed, the percent homology with the human SARS-CoV-2 dropped to 91.5 percent—less than the 93.7 percent shared with the RmYN02 virus detected in bats in China, she said. Wacharapluesadee presented a phylogenetic tree of the complete genome that indicates that RacCS203, a virus found in Thai horseshoe bats, is a new member of the SARS-CoV-2-related coronavirus lineage.

According to a receptor-binding function study on the Thai virus RacCS203 using the phylogenetic tree of the receptor binding domain

(RBD) gene, Wacharapluesadee said it was found to belong to the non-angiotensin converting enzyme-2 (ACE-2) usage clade. Whereas the bat RaTG13 and the human CoV-2 types of coronaviruses can bind ACE-2, these findings indicate that, currently, RacCS203 is not harmful to humans. Rc-0319 from bats in Japan and CoV in pangolins in China were also found to interact with ACE-2.

Sero-surveillance of COVID-19 was conducted in bats and pangolins, said Wacharapluesadee. Samples collected from the animals were tested with an enzyme-linked immunosorbent assay that measures the levels of neutralizing antibody using a surrogate virus neutralization test. The results for the bat sera, she explained, indicated that four of the 98 samples were positive for interaction with SARS-CoV-2—the human RBD. Two of these, she stated, had an inhibition titer greater than 80 percent. As mentioned, the PCR result was positive for 13 percent of the 100 bats tested. For the pangolin serums, Wacharapluesadee said one in 10 was positive against the SARS-CoV-2 RBD antigen using enzyme-linked immunosorbent assay, with a very high percent similarity, as seen in the bat serum. All pangolin samples were PCR negative.

Wacharapluesadee highlighted key findings from this research:

- Serology will be a key tool in performing frontline surveillance.
- Other SC2r-CoV viruses are circulating in bats, and the neutralizing antibodies reflect past infection(s) by other CoV(s) that may be more closely genetically related to SARS-CoV-2.
- More surveillance in animals is needed.

She concluded by noting the impact of multi-sectoral engagement on sentinel surveillance, referral laboratory networking, data sharing, research networking, technology transfer, and policy advice. Moreover, the contributions and collaborations of a wide variety of organizations strengthen the capabilities of the laboratory, enabling it to address novel viruses.

COVID-19 RESPONSE: LESSONS LEARNED TO REINFORCE THE RELEVANCE OF ONE HEALTH PRINCIPLES

Presented by Thierry Nyatanyi, Africa CDC

Nyatanyi outlined existing frameworks for responding to disease outbreaks. He described trade measures the East African region took in response to the COVID-19 pandemic, then detailed Rwanda's government-led, coordinated pandemic response, which included mitigation measures, free medical services, increased production of needed supplies, and vaccine deployment. He also highlighted Rwanda's rapid scale-up of SARS-CoV-2 testing and epidemiology surveillance and listed strategies to improve health system resilience.

Existing Frameworks to Support National Response to Infectious Disease Threats

Nyatanyi explained that numerous regulations are in place to support countries responding to disease outbreaks, such as the World Health Organization's International Health Regulations (WHO's IHR), the World Organisation for Animal Health's (OIE's) Aquatic Animal Health Code and Terrestrial Animal Health Code, and the Tripartite Guide.[5,6,7] Such regulations have informed frameworks that include the IHR monitoring and evaluation framework, national action plans for health security formed through WHO's Joint External Evaluation,[8] OIE's Performance of Veterinary Services Pathway (PVS),[9] IHR-PVS national bridging workshops,[10] and Global Health Security Agenda (GHSA).[11] Nyatanyi noted that all of these allude to preventing the spread of infectious diseases without interfering with international trade. For instance, the purpose and scope of the IHR are "to prevent, protect against, control, and provide a public health response to the international spread of disease in ways that are commensurate with and restricted to public health risks, and which avoid unnecessary interference with international traffic and trade" (WHO, 2008b). Both the Aquatic and Terrestrial Animal Health Codes state that these standards should be used "to develop measures for early detection, internal reporting, notification, control, or eradication of pathogenic agents in animals and preventing their spread via international trade in animals and animal products, while avoiding unjustified sanitary barriers to trade" (OIE, 2019a,b).

---

[5] For the Aquatic Animal Health Code from OIE, see https://www.oie.int/en/what-we-do/standards/codes-and-manuals/aquatic-code-online-access (accessed July 7, 2021).

[6] For the Terrestrial Animal Health Code from OIE, see https://www.oie.int/en/what-we-do/standards/codes-and-manuals/terrestrial-code-online-access (accessed July 7, 2021).

[7] The Tripartite refers to WHO, the Food and Agriculture Organization of the United Nations (FAO), and OIE. For more information on the Tripartite Guide, see http://www.fao.org/documents/card/en/c/CA2942EN (accessed July 7, 2021).

[8] For more information on the joint external evaluation process, see https://www.euro.who.int/en/health-topics/health-emergencies/international-health-regulations/monitoring-and-evaluation/joint-external-evaluation-jee#:~:text=The%20JEE%20is%20a%20voluntary,of%20the%20International%20Health%20Regulations (accessed July 7, 2021).

[9] For more information on the PVS capacity-building platform, see https://www.oie.int/en/what-we-offer/improving-veterinary-services/pvs-pathway (accessed July 7, 2021).

[10] For a fact sheet on the IHR-PVS national bridging workshop, see https://extranet.who.int/sph/sites/default/files/document-library/document/Fact%20sheet%20_final_Lite.pdf (accessed July 7, 2021).

[11] For more information on GHSA, see https://ghsagenda.org (accessed July 7, 2021).

East African Regional Response to COVID-19 Outbreak

Despite the existing guidance, it was challenging to find guidance for the specific issues related to COVID-19 in the early days of the pandemic, Nyatanyi noted. The first case in Rwanda was an imported case confirmed on March 14, 2020, and 6 days later, the government responded by closing the land borders and airport (Karim et al., 2021). Because Rwanda is a landlocked nation, the government allowed travel and trade from neighboring countries to continue, Nyatanyi said, and it was discovered that many truck drivers that were tested as they crossed into Rwanda were positive for the virus. The heads of state within the East African community region met and determined that all COVID-19 test results would be accessible to countries within the region, he said. This practice supported the continuation of travel and trade within the regional economic bloc amid the pandemic. Airports reopened in August 2020, with reverse transcription to polymerase chain reaction (PCR) testing (RT-PCR) required for travelers. The land border partially opened in November 2020. Nyatanyi pointed out that in the absence of international guidance framing the reopening process, Rwanda worked to develop solutions as the pandemic evolved. He added that cases imported into the country continued, highlighting the need to review frameworks moving forward.

Rwanda's Emergency Response Framework

Rwanda has long managed public health threats, including the 2009 influenza A H1N1 pandemic and the 2014 Ebola outbreak in West Africa, said Nyatanyi (Nyamusore et al., 2019; Wane et al., 2012). These outbreaks culminated in implementing One Health as an integrated approach (Nyatanyi et al., 2017). Rwandan senior leadership invested substantial time and resources in establishing a One Health framework for responding to outbreaks, he said, noting that much travel and trade takes place between Rwanda and neighboring Uganda and the Democratic Republic of the Congo—two countries that experience outbreaks of viral hemorrhagic fever every 2–3 years. While a One Health coordination mechanism was in place at the onset of the COVID-19 pandemic, Nyatanyi explained that the global impact led the Rwandan Prime Minister's office to establish a framework specific to COVID-19 days before the first case was diagnosed in the country. It uses an expert advisory team composed of academic institutions and development partners who provide guidance on response measures; its components include epidemiology and surveillance, logistics and administration, risk communication, and planning.

Nyatanyi explained that Rwanda's COVID-19 emergency management plan is chaired by high-level decision makers, allowing for fast-tracking response efforts (see Box 3-1). He noted that adherence to mitigation measures was evidenced by use of public hand-washing stations and social distancing at typically crowded public places, such as bus stops. Local government assisted with enforcement of these mitigation efforts. The COVID-19 services Rwanda provided free of charge—including testing, quarantining, and treatment—proved to be very effective in curbing the spread of infection. Nyatanyi emphasized that government lockdowns can become complicated without public buy-in, but the Rwandan government made efforts to build public trust as lockdowns and closures were instituted. Import delays occurred as truck drivers entering Rwanda tested positive for COVID-19 and had to be quarantined and isolated. These import gaps were addressed by efforts to boost local manufacturing. The production of protective equipment and vaccine deployment fast-tracking are other important components of the emergency response efforts that Nyatanyi noted, explaining that the pandemic has exposed challenge areas that were not addressed by the original One Health coordination mechanism. For example, economic issues related to trade and tourism were not considered until the pandemic.

Nyatanyi presented a graph of COVID-19 incidence rates in Rwanda and Kigali, the nation's capital, from June 2020 to February 2021. A surge of cases in Kigali led to a lockdown in January 2021. He emphasized that

---

BOX 3-1
Fast-Tracked COVID-19 Emergency Management Efforts in Rwanda

Fast-tracked emergency management efforts in Rwanda included the following:

- Consistent and unified messaging for adherence to COVID-19 mitigation measures;
- Free services for COVID-19 testing, quarantine, and treatment;
- Building public trust during enforcement of stringent national measures (lockdown, closure of land borders, and airspace);
- Domestic resource mobilization to support COVID-19 response measures;
- Enforcement of non-pharmaceutical public health measures;
- Decentralization of COVID-19 preparedness and response;
- Supporting local manufacturing to boost import gaps;
- Production of basic essential protection equipment (masks, hand sanitizers, etc.); and
- Fast-tracking vaccine readiness and deployment.

SOURCE: Nyatanyi presentation, February 23, 2021.

an effective lockdown requires coordination, management, and communication, using messaging to convince the public of its necessity. Nyatanyi pointed out that 14 days after the lockdown, the city's COVID-19 cases decreased significantly, from a peak 7-day incidence rate of more than 120 per 100,000 population to less than 100 per 100,000.

Expansion of Rwanda's Testing Capacity and Surveillance

Highlighting the national scale-up of testing capacity, Nyatanyi noted that prior to the SARS-CoV-2 outbreak, Rwanda had only two Rotor-Gene PCR cycler machines able to test for the virus. Within 9 months, procurement of testing machines was fast-tracked, resulting in 88 more being made available in locations across the country, he said. Large-scale training was conducted to create a workforce able to use the new machines, and capacity was expanded to include both rapid and PCR testing. Nyatanyi discussed the role of research in optimizing testing capability. Given the considerable expense of RT-PCR testing, he and his colleagues researched a method in which 20 individual samples are pooled and tested with the resources required for one test (Mutesa et al., 2021). At a low prevalence, they were able to accurately identify infected individuals; in higher-prevalence areas, pooling by 10 samples was found to be effective. Nyatanyi emphasized that this method is cost effective in using far fewer resources to test large groups of people. This exemplifies the need for institutions to work with people on the forefront of service provision to develop innovative ideas, he stated, and pooling is enabling Rwanda to test greater numbers of people at a capacity of 4,000–5,000 tests per day with limited resources.

In addition to testing, Rwanda is using a number of capacity indicators to track virus incidence, including the proportion of hospital beds and intensive care unit beds occupied by COVID-19 patients and the number of home-based care patients with the virus. He noted that Rwanda also tracks the proportion of new cases who have completed contact lists and the proportion of those new contacts that have been notified. While some of these epidemiologic surveillance and capacity indicators are similar to those used by WHO, others are unique to Rwanda, developed while generating solutions for tracking at the country level using geolocation. Rwanda, he explained, has established a four-level alert system with thresholds associated with each indicator—for example, if a given number of people in a village test positive for COVID-19 within a 7-day time frame, that number will determine whether the village is at the "new normal" level or at the low-, moderate-, or high-alert level.

Rwanda's concept architecture for epidemiologic surveillance uses the ArcGIS Enterprise platform for tracking indicators within administrative boundaries, Nyatanyi said, noting that it is an innovative solution created by young engineers.[12] It provides information such as numbers of confirmed cases and deaths by district, age, and gender distributions, as well as whether cases are imported or local. All people have access to this information, including epidemiologists, decision makers, and the general public. The Rwandan government has relied on these data to determine needed efforts in various districts. Furthermore, a number of innovative, homegrown technologies and solutions (e.g., mobile apps for contact tracing) have been developed locally in Rwanda. Nyatanyi stated that innovation is a key area of the pandemic response that can be applied to strengthening One Health implementation.

Improving Health System Resilience

Prior to the COVID-19 pandemic, response reviews typically took place after the end of an outbreak, said Nyatanyi. In an effort to assist countries in reviewing best practices while in the midst of responding to an outbreak, WHO has issued guidance for conducting intra-action reviews (IARs) (WHO, 2020). In Rwanda, Nyatanyi said, IAR has proved to be a valuable tool—particularly during the country's surge of new cases in November 2020—because it was used to update and validate the COVID-19 Strategic Preparedness and Response Plan. IAR also provided Rwanda with insights about gaps, which were identified in all aspects of the response and related to the decentralization of efforts. These included case management, risk communication, coordination, and overwhelmed health facilities. Rwanda also adopted WHO's guidance for home-based care, which required the support of the entire health care system. Community health workers assisted in implementing the approach, which decongested health facilities and assured continuity of health services. Nyatanyi suggested the development of specific One Health metrics for IAR processes while responding to an outbreak.

Nyatanyi stated that lessons learned from Rwanda's government-led approach to COVID-19 can be applied to institutionalizing One Health (see Box 3-2). Emphasizing the value of applying lessons learned from the pandemic to future outbreaks, Nyatanyi closed with the long-standing axiom: "never let a good crisis go to waste."

---

[12] ArcGIS is a software that combines location, map, and analytics data, among others. For more information, see https://www.esri.com/en-us/arcgis/about-arcgis/overview (accessed July 7, 2021).

> **BOX 3-2**
> **Lessons Learned from Rwanda's COVID-19 Response**
>
> - High-level decision making, with government commitment and ownership of setting the agenda, can enable rapid implementation.
> - Fast-tracked legislation and relevant mechanisms can be used to operationalize emergency operation centers and institutionalize One Health.
> - Domestic investments—both government funded and from government partners—can strengthen health systems and potentially fast-track One Health via implementation of Global Health Security Agenda country plans and improvement of WHO Joint External Evaluation scores.
> - Leveraging existing preparedness and response frameworks can ensure continuity of cross-border travel and trade during a pandemic through regional economic blocs.
> - Homegrown innovative approaches can strengthen preparedness and response, including innovation in research and technology.
> - Organizational learning can improve health system resilience by conducting risk analyses and simulations.
> - Investments in research can help to inform policy decisions.
>
> SOURCE: Nyatanyi presentation, February 23, 2021.

DISCUSSION

Funding and Capacity-Building Advocacy

Kester noted that Wiltz-Beckham discussed a comprehensive health department with inter-digitations in multiple areas. While a government's primary role is to ensure the population's safety—and health and public health are indeed aspects of safety—competition for resources from areas such as infrastructure can push public health concerns to the background outside of crises, he said. Given that local and state governments can serve as laboratories of innovation and best practices and that leadership drives resource allocation and capacity building, Kester asked how a public health agency can keep health issues at the forefront of leaders' concerns in the midst of competing needs. Wiltz-Beckham emphasized that all public health efforts require buy-in. Social networking can be used by developing relationships with leaders and even capitalizing on mutual acquaintances who may have their ear. In advocating for public health initiatives, public health practitioners must believe in the work and effectively explain what they do and how and why they do it. Issues of funding and capacity need to be communicated to policy makers, she asserted, as agencies may not meet criteria for grant funding. This is an area of improvement for public health practitioners, and it involves an ongoing process that takes time, Wiltz-Beckham remarked. She gave the example that HCPH had an innovative and forward-thinking leader who traveled to other agencies to learn and share ideas, then brought ideas back to HCPH and led brainstorming sessions around potential benefits and methods of instituting the ideas at their health department. This approach enabled HCPH to fully digest new ideas; in turn, this demonstrated and promoted the importance of One Health to their governing body. Wiltz-Beckham noted that this process can become political, given the role of local, state, and federal government in funding, but that should not discourage public health practitioners from continuing the positive momentum the COVID-19 pandemic has initiated.

Disseminating Best Practices and Innovations

Noting a worldwide need for access to best practices and innovations in addressing the COVID-19 pandemic, Kester asked Nyatanyi whether Rwanda has been able to effectively disseminate information to neighboring countries, given the differences in governments, culture, and language. Nyatanyi replied that academic institutions are channels for conveying information to the scientific community via evidence-based publications and that Rwanda has thusly shared best practices. Sharing innovations regarding information and communications technology has been more challenging, which could be addressed by developing methods of doing so through scientific forums and research institutions, he suggested.

Research Initiative Funding

Kester noted that Wacharapluesadee and her colleagues were able to respond to the evolving COVID-19 pandemic rapidly and comprehensively. He asked whether the initiatives she has been involved in are funded by the government, academia, government–academic partnerships, or external entities; he also queried how she was able to quickly access funding. Wacharapluesadee responded that substantial support for research at the onset of the pandemic in early 2020 came from private-sector donations. These included machines that expanded testing capacity, as the original capacity was only 200–300 cases per day. International support provided the donation of a sequencer. She added that the government also reimburses academic institutions for other research-related costs.

Highlighting the size of Harris County's population and the scope of HCPH's programming, Kester asked Wiltz-Beckham if all efforts rely on government funding or other funding sources are used. She replied that the majority of HCPH's efforts are via general funds and grants from the government. In addition, she explained HCPH has partnered with Latinx faith-based and non-profit organizations to address issues such as lack of access to nutritious food or COVID-19 tests in Houston's large Latinx communities.[13]

Addressing Cultural Attitudes

Noting that Wiltz-Beckham commented on partnering with specific groups who are aware of societal norms, perspectives, and helpful approaches particular to a certain population, Kester asked whether cultural attitudes or traditional health practices played a role in Rwanda's response to the pandemic. Nyatanyi remarked that misperceptions regarding COVID-19 have been common during the pandemic, but Rwanda has worked to identify mechanisms and channels to address misconceptions. The country's Ministry of Health (MOH) recognizes traditional medicine and has an association of registered traditional healers. Thus, traditional healers are part of the health care system and have regular and frequent encounters with ministry personnel. This relationship has established trust and enabled effective communication among MOH, traditional healers, and people treated with traditional medicine, he said, allowing the MOH to dispel misconceptions.

Hypotheses on the Origin of COVID-19

Given the extensive assessments Wacharapluesadee has done thus far, Kester asked for her opinion as to the origin of COVID-19, noting that the risk for other viruses to jump from animals to humans will not disappear with the pandemic. Wacharapluesadee replied that based on her 6 months of study in Thailand during the past year, in which a virus related to SARS-CoV-2 was found in both bats and pangolins, one of these animals was believed to be the progenitor of the virus that evolved and was transmitted to a human and then from human to human. She added that more surveillance is needed to clearly understand all of the SARS-CoV-2-related viruses in animals and arrive at a definitive answer to this question.

One Health Education and Awareness Efforts

Many of the initiatives highlighted during the workshop involve transdisciplinary efforts that developed with the support of external funding

---

[13] The term "Latinx" is a gender-neutral, pan-ethnic label that has been used by some as an alternative to Latino/Latina. For more information, see https://www.pewresearch.org/hispanic/2020/08/11/about-one-in-four-u-s-hispanics-have-heard-of-latinx-but-just-3-use-it (accessed July 7, 2021).

from responsive leadership or coalitions of organizations, said Kester. He posited that One Health's continued growth can be strengthened by developing the concept in medical and veterinary students, thus equipping them with a One Health perspective before they graduate. Noting the impact that providing curricula about recycling in U.S. high schools in years past had on raising teenagers' awareness of recycling, Kester asked the panelists how One Health concepts can be inculcated through the education system. Wiltz-Beckham suggested that efforts begin earlier than postsecondary school, in primary grades. She noted that education efforts about smoking have led children to encourage their family members to give up cigarettes. She added that public health institutions can learn from animal rights organizations, such as People for the Ethical Treatment of Animals, that have used effective marketing strategies to raise awareness. Educating young children means that messages will already be instilled in them when they become future leaders, said Wiltz-Beckham. Kester remarked that educating children about the importance of public health expands on the concept of local jurisdictions serving as laboratories of innovation.

Nyatanyi commented that education efforts need to begin with shifting the mindset of the educators themselves. He noted that while he was leading a One Health steering committee in Rwanda, prominent scholars were unable to agree with one another. When educators disagree, it becomes difficult to translate messaging into academia, he posited. Nyatanyi added that the "brain-drain" phenomenon is an additional challenge Rwanda faces, as youth who are receiving training in school may not remain in the country to apply those learnings as future leaders.

Wacharapluesadee stated that Thailand has a One Health coordinating unit, which is a collaborative effort among seven ministries and the Thai Red Cross. This unit brings the concept of One Health to the community level through health volunteers. She said that in order for communities to be prepared for any emerging infectious disease, training and education are needed. In Thailand, this service is performed by more than 10,000 volunteers and is one mechanism for instilling the One Health concept in the community, said Wacharapluesadee.

Implementing One Health in Underresourced Areas

Kester discussed global disparities in public health and stated that areas lacking in economic growth, infrastructure, and education face challenges in pushing new initiatives forward. He asked Wiltz-Beckham how the best practices developed and continually refined by HCPH can be adopted in places with fewer resources. She replied that public health entities can perform internal scans of their resources and their understanding of the One Health concept. Not all local public health departments look the same, but they all provide some essential public health services. For instance, a local health organization in a rural area may immunize children and perform health inspections at restaurants, she said. Even within this limited scope, opportunities exist to empower people with knowledge. Additionally, opportunities to advocate for One Health can arise while offering current services. For example, she explained, a sanitarian performing inspections may see tires in which mosquitoes are breeding and locate a community partner to provide funding for mosquito dumps. Wiltz-Beckham added that some organizations may be performing One Health work and not even realize it.

Now that HCPH has positions dedicated to carrying forth One Health initiatives, the responsibility to share knowledge and experience with others is incorporated into their roles, Wiltz-Beckham noted. Through mentoring and "training the trainer," HCPH One Health professionals are able to conduct virtual sessions with public health workers in other states and countries. Similar to the counseling South Korea and China have offered other nations regarding COVID-19, best practices can be shared in these sessions, said Wiltz-Beckham. Kester stated that there is good knowledge available, but the challenge lies in disseminating it in the proper context.

Interdepartmental Collaboration

Kester asked Wacharapluesadee for her thoughts on an intergovernmental One Health panel assembled to weave best practices and scientific considerations into policy that can be customized for regional and national considerations. She responded that in Thailand, One Health practice in the government is quite strong. The MOH, DDC, the Department of Livestock Development, and the Department of National Parks, Wildlife, and Plant Conservation work closely together. Research work connects them. For example, in Wacharapluesadee's 10 years of work with the PREDICT project testing novel viruses, a mechanism was in place to report findings to all government sectors. Academic research serves as a tool that draws sectors together in collaborative learning. She remarked that government officers have routine work that prevents them from having time to dedicate to developing the One Health concept, and researchers can connect while working together in offices.

REFLECTIONS FROM DAY 1

Eva Harris, professor of infectious diseases and director of the Center for Global Public Health at the University of California, Berkeley, summarized the day's sessions. She highlighted Goosby's emphasis on establishing transparent, safe spaces in which experts and officials can alert the international community when a threat is detected. Harris also summarized the case studies presented on current One Health initiatives, noting that Rwanda has embraced a One Health approach at the national level for many years; this was evidenced in its multi-sectoral response to the COVID-19 pandemic, in which various ministries have collaborated. Rwanda's multilevel approach has emphasized solutions and innovations from the local to national levels.

Kester discussed several themes that emerged during the first day of the workshop. He noted the key aspects of pandemic prevention highlighted by Goosby: detection, response, and prevention. Whether those areas are placed within the context of a One Health rubric or public health in general, they fit together to form imperatives for public health practitioners and decision makers responsible for keeping the population safe. He also pointed out several themes that arose during the second session's presentations. The first theme is that One Health requires multidisciplinary coordination, which may develop organically but more often must be established with effort and intention. This coordination is needed regardless of whether the setting is a large urban county health department in Texas, a national surveillance and detection effort in Thailand, or a broad public health response to the COVID-19 pandemic in Rwanda. Developing and maintaining coordination can be a challenging endeavor and necessitates constant sustainment, said Kester.

The second theme is the transdisciplinary nature of One Health, involving vectors, vector control, zoonosis, environmental impact, public health, health care systems, education, and more. Kester noted that One Health is not owned by professionals; rather, it is a partnership between professionals, paraprofessionals, and the community. He added that education efforts extended to primary school students could highlight the value of the multidisciplinary aspects of One Health. The third theme is the need for capacity, which underlies the ability to execute ideas, surveil, and prevent and respond to outbreaks. The fourth theme is innovation. Many of the innovations discussed were developed by necessity in response to COVID-19 or as methods of reaching specific populations, said Kester. Innovation applies to laboratory science and also extends to approaches to populations or policy that have never been tried before. He added that many of the innovative practices presented are suitable for greater dissemination regionally and beyond.

The final theme highlighted—perhaps the most important, from Kester's perspective—was touched on by Goosby and in all the presentations: leadership. A well-functioning public health organization cannot be well positioned to anticipate or respond to a crisis if leadership is unaware of that organization's role. Enlightened, educated leadership is needed to prepare for crises, especially given the multiple, competing demands on attention.

Kester remarked that the COVID-19 pandemic remained the global focus, with the reemergence of Ebola in Africa in early 2021 receiving little attention. Public leaders and policy makers can easily divert their attention to other issues, he noted, so strong leadership is needed to make better decisions regarding One Health or public health, which are intertwined.

4

Current One Health Efforts and Opportunities

The first half of the workshop's second session consisted of two panel discussions focused on current One Health initiatives and gaps to address. The moderators began by directly engaging the panelists with questions. The objectives of the discussions were to (1) assess the current status of developing a One Health workforce to identify gaps between employment needs and education and training programs; (2) explore frameworks to establish cross-sector collaborations and community engagement to strengthen threat surveillance and detection; and (3) discuss challenges of and methods for introducing One Health ideology into existing systems for epidemiological surveillance at the local, national, and international levels.

WHAT IS BEING DONE NOW?

Mark Smolinski, president at Ending Pandemics, moderated the first panel discussion, which focused on current applications of the One Health approach. Esron Karimuribo, professor at Sokoine University, Tanzania, discussed community-based data collection efforts. James Hospedales, executive director at the Caribbean Public Health Agency, noted various environmental impacts on pandemic activity and other health considerations and discussed environmental surveillance. David Rizzo, department chair of plant pathology at the University of California, Davis, outlined multiple ramifications of plant health on global health. David Goldman, chief medical officer of the U.S. Food and Drug Administration's (FDA's) Office of Food Policy and Response, addressed the relevance of foodborne illnesses. Carrie S. McNeil, One Health specialist at Ending Pandemics, described simulations in preparedness efforts.

AfyaData Tool and Experience from Tanzania

Smolinski asked about the One Health community-based surveillance approach developed in Thailand, which was replicated in Tanzania with the AfyaData tool, which is an app with web and mobile components intended to facilitate collection of data regarding human and animal health events at the community level and make it available at national and global levels.[1] Karimuribo explained that the approach was community focused from the outset. During the design process, officials working with human and animal populations were brought together with the community to identify surveillance challenges. The AfyaData participatory disease surveillance technology factored in these challenges during development for use at the community level as part of a One Health approach. This community focus incorporates the local environment, including local languages. The AfyaData system was designed for use by both community members and community health workers, so it needed to be multilingual, enabling users to feel comfortable identifying and reporting events regardless of language. The brand name for the technology is rooted in this community focus: "afya" is the Swahili word for "health." Karimuribo shared a visual representation of AfyaData.[2] Karimuribo and his colleagues have proposed a vision of a unified, verified signal that is shared by numerous ministries that deal with health, livestock, wildlife, and environment. It would enable these actors to see events unfolding in real time and generate information to inform their responses.

Support from the United States enabled Tanzania to establish a One Health coordination desk at the Office of the Prime Minister, which also houses the Disaster Management Department, Karimuribo explained. These improvements facilitate managing disease outbreaks, mobilizing human and financial resources, and deploying support staff for verification and diagnosis. For instance, the AfyaData tool was used successfully by a community-level One Health reporter in Ulanga, Tanzania, who reported a sudden rise in dog bites. The tool enabled rapid response mobilization, whereby an outbreak of rabies was confirmed and followed by immediate containment measures, including mass dog vaccination and awareness efforts. This exemplifies how AfyaData links data from community events with officials who can initiate responses.

Smolinski noted Karimuribo's engagement with the Maasai community in Tanzania while designing the AfyaData tool. The proximity of

---

[1] An outline comparing the two systems can be found here: https://www.exemplars.health/emerging-topics/epidemic-preparedness-and-response/surveillance-technology-ending-pandemics-case-study (accessed May 30, 2021).

[2] More information about the Afyadata tool can be found at http://afyadata.sacids.org (accessed April 29, 2021).

the Maasai community's livestock to wildlife, nature preserves, and parks caused some concern among international partners about the potential for spillover from wildlife into the domestic animal population. Smolinski asked whether engagement with the Maasai community or its use of the data-sharing tool has led to behavioral changes. Karimuribo replied that the community was first engaged during the initial design of the AfyaData system. In asking them about the challenges they faced, it was discovered that the community was concerned about water sources as a potential point of disease transmission between humans and animals. Ngorongoro is a world heritage site with a unique ecosystem that is cohabitated by humans, wild animals, and domestic animals. Using input from the Maasai community, a system was designed to support the control of human and animal diseases. Karimuribo reported that after 10 years in operation, the system has brought about behavioral changes, particularly with respect to how the community responds to the system's reports. Multiple community-level events involving schoolchildren and abnormal primate behavior have been identified, linked to wildlife, investigated, and contained.

Impacts of Human Destruction of Nature on Global Health

Smolinski asked about the impact of human destruction of nature, such as deforestation, and other ecosystem disturbances on the emergence of new diseases. Hospedales stated that over the past 40 years, most pandemics have emerged out of forests and wetlands encroached upon by human activities, such as agriculture and legal and illegal logging. This ecological pressure and displacement of animals from their habitats can promote pandemics and is linked to larger concerns of climate change and degradation of environments. The One Health initiative could gain traction by connecting to the broader climate consciousness that is growing among governments, businesses, and even celebrities and popular culture, said Hospedales. Deforestation is associated with loss of biodiversity and the release of carbon dioxide into the atmosphere, which in turn creates hospitable conditions for pandemics. Thus, slowing and halting forest destruction could be beneficial in terms of pandemic control. Moreover, areas of forest being destroyed could be targets of increased surveillance efforts, including satellite-based systems[3] combined with collecting on-the-ground syndromic data from pharmacies and health centers to produce an early warning system for pandemics. Rather than waiting for the first case of a new pandemic virus to occur, Hospedales asserted, such an early warning system could look at the confluence of circumstances that lead to pandemics.

---

[3] Hospedales gave the example of Planet: https://www.planet.com (accessed May 30, 2021).

Although plants are an important part of the environment, they are often ignored in discussions of pandemics, said Smolinski. He asked about the relevance of plant pathogens to broader considerations of pandemic control. Rizzo commented on the role of plant health within the One Health framework. Food security and food availability are reliant upon plant health, which can be adversely affected by insects, biotic and abiotic agents, and plant pathogens. Food safety is a major concern linked to One Health, Rizzo explained, because vegetable crops can be contaminated by wild and domesticated animals that harbor human pathogens such as *E. coli* and *Salmonella*. Rizzo noted a few examples of the interface between plant and human health. Mycotoxins (toxic secondary metabolites caused by some fungi that infect plants) are capable of causing disease and death in humans and other animals. Plant diseases can also have economic impacts. For instance, coffee is not a staple crop, but coffee farming provides livelihoods for millions of people in low-income countries. The emergence of coffee rust disease in Central America destroyed many coffee crops and caused indirect adverse health effects for residents. Moreover, the impacts of deforestation extend beyond destroying trees to include spreading plant pathogens and insects. Deforestation and the export of commodities harvested from forests have introduced exotic species and pathogens to new environments, contributing to global One Health concerns. These factors are interlinked, with plant health as one nexus of these linkages. Rizzo pointed out that the majority of all food comes from plants, either directly or indirectly, through animal feed. Because plant health is a major component of One Health, he suggested that pathologists should collaborate with plant health researchers to pursue the One Health approach.

Food and the One Health Approach

Smolinski noted that despite the relevance of foodborne illnesses to One Health, they are often omitted from initiatives and instead addressed as a siloed issue. He asked how foodborne illnesses can be incorporated into a broader conception of One Health. Goldman remarked that his experience in the U.S. Department of Agriculture (USDA) food safety and inspection service and his nearly 20 years working on foodborne illness at FDA have given him insight into these issues. The interplay of animals, environment, and human health has long been evident, yet this interplay has only been considered within the context of One Health in recent years. For example, the initiation of PulseNet in the mid-1990s by the U.S. Centers for Disease Control and Prevention (CDC) and other partners involved comparing unique genetic characteristics of food samples, environmental samples, and human clinical isolates.[4] These comparisons linked foodborne illness with the exposure that caused the disease. Since then, whole-genome sequencing has become a powerful surveillance tool for comparing the genetic characteristics of food, environment—either the natural environment or the food manufacturing environment—and human illness, he added.

Goldman noted that the National Center for Biotechnology Information at the National Institutes of Health (NIH) has a catalog of more than 500,000 pathogens, including bacterial pathogens that may link human illness with environmental and animal pathogens, which enables federal officials to look daily for links between illness and pathogens, which can be confirmed using epidemiology. This process can enable early identification of an outbreak, affording the opportunity to respond quickly to prevent secondary cases. The interplay of humans, food animals, wild animals, environments, and crops warrants more exploration. Goldman noted that researchers have focused on this interplay of pathogens and the environments and ecologies in which they live, thrive, and become available to cause human infections.

Using Outbreak Simulations to Promote One Health Readiness

Smolinski remarked that Sandia National Laboratories have been instrumental in developing simulation exercises—often referred to as "tabletop exercises"—to improve One Health efforts. He asked how this methodology is used to strengthen national programs and regional collaboration. McNeil said that emergency management actors have long used simulations to improve readiness and strengthen preparedness for various types of outbreaks and emergencies. When assessing One Health readiness, it is clear that ecosystem health, plant health, public health, and animal health are studied in siloed fields; these fields' bodies of knowledge are siloed accordingly. This disconnection between sectors is detrimental to the early stages of outbreak detection as well as the response stages. Intended to mimic real-life conditions, simulations can be used to identify and address the barriers created by silos.

Sandia National Laboratories has developed role-based multiplayer, multi-scenario exercises with participant-led analysis, said McNeil. These exercises put participants in roles similar to those they would likely play during a real outbreak. In 2015, Sandia, on behalf of Ending Pandemics, coordinated an exercise in South Asia with One Health participants from 13 ministries across eight countries, each with a unique scenario. The focus

---

[4] PulseNet is a national surveillance network for foodborne illnesses that was originally established to collect molecular subtyping data from pulse field gel electrophoresis analysis, accessible at https://www.cdc.gov/pulsenet/index.html (accessed May 30, 2021).

was to test cross-sector, cross-border coordination during an emerging novel coronavirus. Epidemiologists and public health workers focused on public health data, case definitions, and line lists; laboratorians (individuals who work in laboratories) were faced with everyday challenges, such as freezer space and incoming samples. Simulation participants are only provided information that someone in their role would be privy to in real life. For example, public health workers are not given data from the animal health sector, because in a real outbreak, the public health sector would not have access to that information. McNeil explained that by testing these systems through simulations, participants are able to analyze for themselves where information sharing and coordination are taking place, where they are lacking, and where they could be improved upon.

In the exercise conducted in South Asia, Sandia National Laboratories and Ending Pandemics looked at cross-sector collaboration between the animal health and public health sectors and cross-border collaboration among all countries, said McNeil. Participants identified the need for a South Asia One Health disease surveillance network to foster information sharing across borders. Since then, additional remote and in-person simulation exercises have informed the development of the South Asia One Health disease surveillance network. One of these activities was to use simulations to inform disease prioritization for the network. The multirole, multi-scenario approach to conducting exercises used at the regional level has also been applied to national initiatives. Numerous countries have received training in this methodology through Biothreat Readiness Leadership trainings. McNeil explained that Sandia National Laboratories offers the Portal for Readiness Exercises and Planning (PREP), a free, online software platform that tracks information and multiple scenarios related to biothreats.[5] Biothreat readiness leaders have tested their national One Health strategies with tabletop exercises and also conducted exercises at operational levels, such as in response to outbreaks of Rift Valley fever and brucellosis. She highlighted several opportunities that outbreak simulations can provide: (1) building relationships in advance of an outbreak, a component she identified as critical for successful outbreak response; (2) fostering appreciation for each sector's strengths and unique challenges; and (3) developing specific plans for how to move forward.

---

[5] More information about PREP can be found at https://gcbs.sandia.gov/tools/prep.html (accessed April 29, 2021). Ending Pandemics hosts its own version of this multiplayer tabletop exercise software, called "START$_x$," which can be located at https://endingpandemics.org/startx-exercises (accessed July 28, 2021).

Integrating Environmental Surveillance Within Public Health Systems

Smolinski asked how environmental surveillance can be better integrated into public health. Hospedales acknowledged the importance of this and pointed out that the tendency toward compartmentalization can complicate responses to even simple outbreaks, referring to his experience in CDC's Epidemiology Intelligence Service investigating shigellosis caused by eggs. In some countries, aspects of environmental surveillance have been internalized effectively. For example, in Trinidad and Tobago, the ministry recently issued a note indicating that numerous monkeys had been found dead in the southern forests. Presumptive causes of death for New World monkeys include lead poisoning and yellow fever. Therefore, this type of event can serve as an early warning for a yellow fever outbreak, which can be addressed with a vaccination campaign. Such a response exemplifies an effective integration of environmental surveillance into public health systems. Furthermore, digital health technology affords innovative possibilities, Hospedales noted. For instance, citizens and health workers can use mobile phones to take measurements for powerful environmental surveillance. The increasing access to digital tools, along with the growing interest in environmental surveillance, can strengthen the integration of environmental surveillance within public health systems.

Applying Plant Pathology to Human and Animal Diseases

Smolinski remarked that plants can serve as a model system to advance knowledge or methods that are directly applicable to human health; he asked Rizzo to expound upon this perspective of plant health. Rizzo said that many of the processes that occur in humans and animals also occur in plants. Although there are clear differences between plants and humans, specific concepts from plant pathogen research can be applied to humans and animals (e.g., aerial pathogen surveillance, innate immunity). Moreover, plant research is not constrained by certain ethical considerations that apply to humans and animals. Finally, he pointed out that plant pathologists work with units of population and community, not individual plants. For example, an individual wheat plant has little value and is not the focus. Thus, plant pathologists can offer modeling and community epidemiology insights and skills.

Using Whole-Genome Sequencing in the One Health Approach

Smolinski noted that whole-genome sequencing has revolutionized disease surveillance. He asked how this technology can be applied broadly to help advance the One Health approach. Goldman remarked that whole-genome sequencing provides the opportunity to make connections at the molecular genetics level. Traditional epidemiological processes are then used to verify that the connections are in fact related to exposures that caused illness. This combination of processes holds great promise for advancing foodborne illness surveillance, said Goldman. He emphasized that the power of whole-genome sequencing lies in its capacity to reveal connections in real time. Each day, federal and state officials query an expansive database to identify these connections, yielding early warnings about potential outbreaks and facilitating quick and early responses.

Using Simulation Technology During the COVID-19 Pandemic

Smolinski asked how Sandia National Laboratories has applied their simulation technology to the COVID-19 pandemic. McNeil replied that each outbreak or simulation would ideally conclude with an after-action review to evaluate the actions taken and identify opportunities for improvement. Needed changes are then identified and implemented into future plans and training resources. However, in the midst of the COVID-19 outbreak, it has been challenging to create opportunities for such reflection. Because reflection is critical, Ending Pandemics and Sandia have developed a during-action review and tabletop (DART) methodology, said McNeil. This approach incorporates a prospective element, rather than just retrospective reflection, and identifies how future scenarios can be used to address concerns of communities and countries. DART allows participants to consider the information needed today to best prepare for potential events in the near or distant future. As the One Health paradigm applies to the COVID-19 pandemic, the simulation incorporates a One Health perspective.

McNeil remarked that One Health strengths can be called upon in situations that warrant a high level of surge capacity. For example, the animal health and plant health sectors have polymerase chain reaction (PCR) testing capabilities, and animal health workers are trusted community members who contribute in valuable ways to risk communication in the field. The plant health and animal health sectors have numerous capabilities—ranging from logistics to epidemiology to laboratory to emergency management—and this capacity can be leveraged across other sectors. McNeil added that such cross-sector leveraging has been implemented during the COVID-19 pandemic. Thus, an opportunity exists to sustain such activities and develop institutional policies that strengthen and improve resource sharing and surge capacity. She noted that challenges have arisen when animal health workers could not access personal protective equipment due to the increase in demand caused by COVID-19. This challenge presents an opportunity to plan for such occasions by creating stockpiles for them. Other mitigation strategies can be considered, such as obtaining supplies from universities or schools. While it is impossible to accurately predict the worst-case scenario that will become reality, simulation scenarios can help to identify opportunities to mitigate and prepare for potential situations.

Smolinski asked whether the simulations use virtual reality training. McNeil responded that the ones she discussed are strategic, operational policy-level simulations that can reveal how well participants are coordinating and working together. Sandia National Laboratories has developed other video-game-based simulations for tactical level trainings, such as carcass disposal and waste management tasks. She noted that simulations using video game technology can improve readiness in underresourced communities that may be unable to send staff for hands-on One Health emergency training. Sandia has also explored virtual reality and augmented reality technologies. While it would be possible to develop simulations using these technologies, they have opted not to do so thus far, said McNeil. In developing the PREP platform, Sandia discovered the benefits of keeping its training modules as simple as possible and requiring minimal bandwidth. She acknowledged promising and interesting opportunities to use virtual reality and augmented reality in training simulations, such as those for biosafety and biosecurity training. However, the current need is best met with simpler, more immediately available technology, she contended.

Protecting Environments Using the One Health Approach

Smolinski asked whether community-based tools or other components of the One Health approach are helping to conserve ecological integrity. Karimuribo noted that AfyaData can be adapted for any scenario. For example, some districts in Tanzania had concerns related to environmental health, so the tool was adapted to support data collection related to these concerns. Given an existing framework and tools, the AfyaData system can facilitate the digitization of information and link responders to data. Hospedales said research investigating integrated coastal and aquaterrestrial solutions brought about advances for small islands' management of marine protected areas, engagement with farmers, sustainable use of pesticides, and drainage. He posited that the rapid rate of deforestation and wetland destruction could be addressed, at least in part, by improving surveillance for emergent problems and facilitating increased government scrutiny and corporate accountability. Surveillance could be improved by using satellite imagery and high-resolution drone imagery. To that end, a deal has been brokered with the drone pilots' association in Trinidad and Tobago to enlist pilots in supporting continuous surveillance of brushfires and assisting with rapid detection and response. This approach may be beneficial in other settings, such as in Africa, Asia, and the Amazon. Hospedales added that public scrutiny of human-caused environmental destruction may also serve as a deterrent to those who may carry out these activities.

Applying Systems Thinking Approaches in Food Systems

Smolinski asked about the forces at play in communities that rely upon seafood and coastal ecosystems. Hospedales replied that the understudied concept of complexity in ecosystems is relevant to this issue. Numerous environmental factors interconnect, with implications that are not widely appreciated. For example, high levels of Sahara dust are transporting aspergillus spores to coral reefs, and sargassum weed has spread to the point of becoming contiguous from West Africa to the Western Atlantic Ocean. These types of large-scale events exemplify interconnected factors that should be studied, said Hospedales. Although researchers may be skilled at reductionist science, they are often less adept at studying how factors are interconnected, he added. Rizzo further elaborated that, similar to the concerning rise of antimicrobial resistance (AMR) among bacterial pathogens, the overuse of fungicides may have effects that can spill over into fungal diseases among humans that can be particularly concerning for those with compromised immune systems. This is yet another example of the interconnections between systems and the need for widespread information sharing and collaboration. McNeil maintained that a systems approach should be applied when considering any food system. In addition to the large-scale interconnected factors, the downstream effects on communities should also be considered, including immediate food security and subsequent health issues and risks.

Integrating One Health with National Security

Smolinski noted that in many countries, much of the national budget is allocated to national defense. He asked about strategies to link the One Health mission to national security, in terms of funding and government buy-in, and opportunities for military branches to partner with One Health programs in activities such as deployment and data sharing. Goldman said that from the food safety perspective, the U.S. Department of Defense (DOD) has been a long-time One Health partner. For example, USDA has a National Advisory Committee on Microbiological Criteria for Foods, and DOD has contributed to the knowledge base on foodborne pathogens since the committee's inception.[6] Such efforts contribute to the One Health mission by improving the understanding of connections between foodborne pathogens, exposures, and human illness.

---

[6] The National Advisory Committee on Microbiological Criteria for Foods is currently part of the Food Safety and Inspection Service at the U.S. Department of Agriculture; its executive committee includes liaisons from DOD and other federal agencies. More information can be found at https://www.fsis.usda.gov/policy/advisory-committees/national-advisory-committee-microbiological-criteria-foods-nacmcf (accessed May 30, 2021).

Plant-Based Medicines and One Health

Although not all plant-based medicines have been shown to be effective, much of the world uses these treatments, noted Smolinski. Their use is often culturally determined and is unlikely to be replaced by more expensive drugs. He asked about the role that One Health might play in better understanding the widespread use of these medicines. Acknowledging that he is not a plant-medicine expert, Rizzo noted that traditional medicines extend beyond plants to include fungi, such as mushrooms. Many plants clearly have medicinal properties, as important medicines have been derived from plants for centuries. From the One Health standpoint, the study of plant medicine should be approached with an open mind, he added. Collaboration with anthropologists, sociologists, and practitioners of Western medicine can help encourage stakeholders to maintain an attitude of openness about the effectiveness of traditional medicines.

Karimuribo explained that pastoral communities in Tanzania often value the lives of animals above the lives of humans. In these communities, individuals may accept traditional medicine for their own health needs while seeking commercial veterinary products for their animals. This dynamic creates a unique point of entry in these communities. For example, a mass animal vaccination campaign could be used as an opportunity to address human health awareness issues or conduct short human-health screenings.

Crowdsourcing Event Verification

Smolinski asked how Tanzania's community-based approach addresses rumors that move though the system and whether the AfyaData system is integrated or collaborating with data systems such as Program for Monitoring Emerging Diseases (ProMED)-mail[7] or EpiCore.[8] Karimuribo explained that Tanzania's system has a module called "AfyaWatch," which is designed to enlist community members in conducting local-level verification of reported events. Individuals who do so are given a credibility score based on the accuracy of their reports. These scores enable local verifications to link with official verification, reducing the need for ministry officials in the livestock and environmental sectors to verify the events. Furthermore, the Tanzanian systems are being linked with global scanning reports, including ProMED-mail and EpiCore. By integrating local data with global

---

[7] ProMED is a source of information for clinicians and laboratorians, providing timely reporting of pathogens and their vectors. More information is available from https://promedmail.org (accessed March 30, 2021).

[8] Smolinski explained that EpiCore is a crowd-based epidemiology community that volunteers to verify any signal that comes through automated disease surveillance systems. More information is available at https://endingpandemics.org/projects/epicore (accessed March 30, 2021).

data systems within its data science management module, Tanzania can use advanced analytical approaches and artificial intelligence modeling for prediction and intervention.

Integrating the Private Sector into One Health Approaches

Given the private sector's role in environmental health, Smolinski asked how it can become more engaged with One Health challenges. Goldman said that foodborne illness is a One Health problem; therefore, it should be addressed by a One Health solution. For example, discerning the contamination of produce involves understanding how land adjacent to agricultural fields is used. This requires collaboration between numerous private parties, including produce growers, farmers, ranchers, and possibly state authorities. McNeil said that the private sector is critical at every stage of One Health. Private-sector actors contribute initial detection efforts in the livestock industry and beyond, as well as in response activities, including logistics and response equipment supply. She said inclusion of private-sector actors in simulation exercises is one way to develop coordination and trust with the private sector. In an assessment conducted in the United States, they found that more engagement with the private sector is needed to build trust, forge partnerships, and bolster preparedness.

Hospedales raised the issue of private-sector cooperation with military actors in the arena of health security. In the Caribbean, hurricane response efforts have necessitated civilian–military cooperation. However, other regions, such as Central America, may have tension between military and civilian systems. In these settings, fostering civilian–military cooperation for epidemic detection and response initiatives can be challenging. In the Caribbean, presidents have mandated that many federal agencies—including public health and security agencies—work together. The European Union has funded simulations to test how these actors can best collaborate in response to various public health emergencies. Hospedales added that in past decades, a network of U.S. military labs in Cairo, Kenya, and Asia had access to veterinary and animal sources. Data from these types of networks could be integrated with environmental data to good effect, he noted.

In closing, Smolinski highlighted the role of natural history collections and other biological collections in One Health systems. These collections have helped solve challenges with emerging pathogens in the past. The Smithsonian Museum of Natural History currently features the *Outbreak: Epidemics in a Connected World* exhibit, which explores epidemics in an emerging and interconnected world with a One Health lens.[9] The work

---

[9] More information about the *Outbreak: Epidemics in a Connected World* exhibit can be found at https://naturalhistory.si.edu/exhibits/outbreak-epidemics-connected-world (accessed April 29, 2021).

involved in creating this exhibit demonstrates the valuable research that comes from the Smithsonian Natural History Collection, said Smolinski. He suggested that improving natural collection infrastructure in the Global South could be of benefit to others.[10]

OPPORTUNITIES FOR IMPROVEMENT

John Nkengasong, director at the Africa Centres for Disease Control and Prevention, moderated the second panel discussion. Panelists focused on knowledge and dissemination, interfacing mechanisms, policy issues, and strategies to connect the relevance of One Health to sectors beyond the traditional health sectors (e.g., economies, local industries, other stakeholders). John Balbus, senior advisor for public health at the National Institute of Environmental Health Sciences (NIEHS), discussed how data can be used both to improve global health and advance the One Health approach. Christopher Braden, deputy director at the National Center for Emerging and Zoonotic Infectious Diseases, addressed the modernization of surveillance systems and formalization of collaborative partnerships. Carlos Das Neves, president at the International Wildlife Disease Association, highlighted One Health approaches in low-income countries that can serve as exemplary models for higher-income countries. Cristina Romanelli, program officer of biodiversity, climate change, and health at the World Health Organization (WHO), described opportunities for society to shift toward a fairer, healthier, greener civilization in the wake of the COVID-19 pandemic.

Gaps and Challenges in One Health Approaches

Nkengasong asked panelists to speak about challenges facing the United States and other nations, with a focus on identifying areas that are lagging behind in terms of integration into One Health systems. Balbus considered several areas in which challenges have been created by stove-piping—a process in which data are funneled directly to high-ranking authorities. For example, at the 1992 UN Conference on Environment and Development in Rio de Janeiro, Brazil, two conventions were signed pertaining to the domains of biodiversity and climate change.[11] In the decades since, efforts to integrate these domains remain limited. Balbus suggested that this

---

[10] McNeil noted that a Project Echo series was conducted entitled "Museums and Emerging Pathogens in the Americas." More information is available from https://hsc.unm.edu/echo/institute-programs/mepa (accessed March 30, 2021).

[11] The two conventions signed were the Convention on Biological Diversity (see https://www.cbd.int/doc/legal/cbd-en.pdf) and the United Nations Framework Convention on Climate Change (see https://unfccc.int/files/essential_background/background_publications_htmlpdf/application/pdf/conveng.pdf) (both accessed July 7, 2021).

insufficient integration is rooted in the signing of separate conventions, as opposed to a joint convention on biodiversity and climate change. Similarly, vertical agendas within the federal government isolate various domains, such as the Global Health Security Agenda[12] and RBM Partnership to End Malaria.[13] These and other major programs have been initiated to address existing problems, yet environmental health and One Health programs instituted by CDC and other agencies are not often integrated into them. This lack of integration is evidenced by certain executive orders, in which colleagues may call for reviews of the Global Health Security Agenda or mention the impact of climate change, but these concerns are not brought to the fore and the environmental perspective is not fully integrated into the programs. Balbus emphasized that One Health extends beyond pandemics, zoonotic spillover, and animal health. Gaps are evident in oceanic and microbial studies and the One Health–related interconnection of plants, animals, ecosystems, and microbes. These interconnections represent primary mechanisms through which climate change and environmental change will affect the health of all life on Earth.

Braden discussed central issues related to early detection and response and ongoing surveillance challenges. Researchers often struggle to bring together data sources—such as laboratory and epidemiological data—so broadening data collection at the tactical level presents challenges. However, advancements in the conceptualization of data and surveillance are constrained by antiquated systems, he noted. These systems need modernization with updated data architectures and sources, paired with updated technical aspects, such as cloud technology, data pipelines, and integration tools that allow data to be layered in terms of animal, human, and environmental health. New tools are available that may aid in the transition toward more modern data systems. Additionally, better cooperation among agencies would contribute to verifying and investigating reported signals. Conducting investigations within silos can be challenging, and working collaboratively across silos can be even more daunting, but cross-disciplinary approaches are needed at the international, national, state, and local levels, said Braden. For instance, when a domestic foodborne outbreak is detected in the United States, experts in human, environmental, and animal health should collaborate in the investigations.

Das Neves suggested that strengthening One Health systems could begin with developing greater interconnectivity and broadening the focus on health systems to extend to financial, political, and social systems.

---

[12] More information about Global Health Security Agenda is available from https://ghsagenda.org (accessed April 30, 2021).

[13] More information about the RBM Partnership to End Malaria is available from https://endmalaria.org (accessed April 30, 2021).

Countries have been fairly effective at managing AMR and recognizing the need for greater connectivity and transformation in those efforts; however, this recognition has yet to extend to other areas. Politicians, industry, pharmaceutical companies, and other private and public stakeholders from high-income nations have partnered on initiatives in low- and middle-income countries, while efforts in their home countries are less comprehensive. The missing factors in achieving collaboration may include awareness, interaction, interest, funding, and political will. Das Neves noted that Nigeria and Rwanda have national One Health strategic plans, but many higher-income countries do not. Lastly, referencing the Venn diagram often used to represent One Health, he remarked that much attention is given to the overlap of the human, animal, and environmental health circles, but nurturing each of those individual areas often receives inadequate consideration.

Romanelli spoke of the broad, interdisciplinary, global view she has developed through her work on sustainable development, global health policy, biological diversity, and environmental science. She emphasized that a more inclusive and coordinated One Health framework is needed. One Health offers an integrated approach to developing purposeful and coordinated responses to some of the greatest global health, environmental, socioeconomic, and political challenges through the lens of systems thinking. However, it also provides an opportunity for diverse stakeholders to work together across sectors and disciplines to take a preventive role in addressing the root causes of ill health. This approach has the power to tackle interconnected challenges, while also strengthening monitoring, preparedness, and response to future health threats. By building the capacity for prevention, One Health can also help to address the social, environmental, and economic determinants of ill health with equity as a driving force in the context of global environmental change. The COVID-19 pandemic has brought to the fore the interconnectedness between the human, animal, and natural worlds. According to Romanelli, the international community has largely failed to adopt a systems approach to planetary health. While time is limited, progress remains possible. She acknowledged that One Health is not the only interdisciplinary and cross-sectoral approach using a systemic lens—conservation medicine, EcoHealth, and planetary health seek to bring about action in a similar manner. Still, One Health provides a valuable opportunity to governments, the scientific community, the public and private sectors, and local communities to develop robust evidence-based strategies for future action.

Romanelli noted that the COVID-19 pandemic has brought society to a crossroads: decisions about how to rebuild may either perpetuate the damaging economic development patterns and practices of recent decades or bring about progress toward a healthier, fairer, greener civilization. She highlighted WHO's efforts toward the latter, including a comprehensive manifesto launched in July 2020 to chart the path toward a healthy, green, and just recovery from the pandemic.[14] The manifesto calls on the international community to prioritize health recovery and center the issues of biodiversity and climate protection to prepare for and reduce vulnerability to future health emergencies. The manifesto sets forth six prescriptions for a healthy, green recovery that span 80 targeted action areas: (1) protecting and conserving nature, which is the source of human health; (2) investing in essential services, from water and sanitation to clean energy in health care facilities; (3) ensuring a quick, healthy energy transition; (4) promoting healthy, sustainable food systems; (5) building healthy, livable cities; and (6) stopping the use of taxpayer money to fund pollution. Romanelli emphasized that the prescription to protect and preserve nature is the starting point of the other five. Recognizing and protecting nature as the source of human health has largely been absent from the One Health narrative, she noted. As part of its commitment to One Health over the past several decades, WHO has identified the need to adopt a broader perspective that expands beyond the full range of infectious and noncommunicable diseases to encompass the ecological and environmental dimensions. Romanelli noted that developing and implementing One Health programs in past decades has inadequately addressed environmental concerns at national and global levels.

Successful One Health Implementation Efforts

Nkengasong asked for examples of successful implementation of the One Health approach. Das Neves highlighted the PREDICT program, as well as similar efforts established by the European Union. Additionally, several African and Southeast Asian nations have built effective systems with little to no pre-existing architecture. The creation of a new system may help motivate stakeholders and encourage collaboration, he added. Although higher-income countries may already have existing functional systems in place that can address specific issues, they are also prone to siloing. Thus, he suggested that the strongest examples of One Health program implementation at present come from countries that have struggled with disease, environmental conditions, economic problems, and insecure food systems. Rwanda exemplifies the One Health progress that can be achieved in countries facing these intersectional challenges. In comparison, developed nations often lag behind due to political or economic factors or the silos long

---

[14] More information about the WHO Manifesto for a healthy recovery from COVID-19 is available from https://www.who.int/news-room/feature-stories/detail/who-manifesto-for-a-healthy-recovery-from-covid-19 (accessed March 31, 2021).

established in One Health–related sectors. Stakeholders who have worked in siloed fields for decades may be more resistant to collaborative, cross-sector activities than those in countries with newer systems. Das Neves suggested that nations in Europe and North America should also study the accomplishments of countries in Africa to inform their own efforts.

Balbus posited that a predictor for the success of a One Health system may be its sentinel species. Systems using sentinel animal species, such as chickens in agricultural systems, for early detection and surveillance have incorporated fundamental One Health approaches. When the sentinel species is human—including severe acute respiratory syndrome coronavirus 2 and Ebola—the origins of an outbreak often lie in wild rather than agricultural systems. Balbus described the human interface with wild systems as a frontier for the One Health approach. New sensor and technological solutions that can be deployed remotely and on the ground could expand surveillance into this frontier.

Braden noted that One Health approaches have been most successful in places where animal environments and human health are naturally tied together, even to the point of creating unique silos; these types of scenarios lend themselves to an interdigitated approach. For example, rabies control requires dog vaccination programs. Regardless of the label attached to these efforts, they are inherently One Health approaches. The same is true of food safety and vector-borne diseases because effective vector control requires ecological considerations. He added that AMR is a long-standing area of focus for multiple sectors. In recent years, the availability of new funding streams has fueled progress in addressing this issue, with leaders actively engaged in ensuring that a One Health approach was adopted. However, the U.S. national action plan does not address the environmental component. For instance, commonly used pesticides are often antifungals that are important in human medicine, and aspergillus may be gaining resistance to the antifungals used in agriculture. These examples underscore the value of the types of cross-sectoral observations made possible by the One Health approach, said Braden.

Romanelli acknowledged the successes cited by the panel, but she cautioned that now is not the time for celebration or complacency. Excellent work has been achieved, such as the PREDICT program, but much work remains at the local, national, and global scales. At the global level, the tripartite alliance among WHO, the Food and Agriculture Organization of the United Nations (FAO), and the World Organisation for Animal Health (OIE) has revealed areas of failure and weakness.[15] Established to address the gaps in One Health approaches, this alliance found that the ecological

---

[15] More information about the tripartite alliance can be found at https://who.int/foodsafety/areas_work/zoonose/concept-note/en (accessed April 29, 2021).

and environmental dimensions of One Health have largely been ignored, while the human–animal interface has received far greater attention, said Romanelli.

Das Neves added that societal involvement has been valuable in settings where One Health approaches have been successful. Achieving buy-in from veterinarians, doctors, and even politicians is relatively straightforward, but getting buy-in from communities and society can be more challenging, he noted. For example, local businesspeople may need to change their business models, big industry will need to adopt environmental perspectives, and children require education before bad habits are formed. The most successful One Health programs are those that engage all stakeholders with roles to play in One Health solutions, said Das Neves.

Institutionalizing and Formalizing Collaborative Agreements for One Health Approaches

Nkengasong noted that many One Health initiatives have been informal arrangements among committed individuals in separate organizations or departments. He asked how such initiatives can be formalized to foster ongoing collaboration that can be maintained through changes in personnel. In the United States, these initiatives often result from one-on-one relationships, but they need to be institutionalized, said Braden, along with the collaboration and integration they involve. This institutionalization can be challenging, because it requires support from leadership and the creation of charters, cooperative agreements, and memorandums to formalize working relationships. He remarked that no single agreement will adequately establish the needed degree of collaboration, so multiple agreements are often implemented. For example, one formal cooperative relationship was established to facilitate data sharing between FDA, USDA, and CDC. Another formal cooperative relationship aims to promote collaboration in conducting outbreak investigations by establishing standard operating procedures, identifying the roles of each agency, and stating the expectations for outbreak preparedness and response. Other agreements have been created related to the use of molecular data in whole genome sequencing to ensure that all appropriate agencies are involved. In addition to the numerous aspects of cooperation that must be formalized at various levels of the participating institutions, cooperation also needs to be formalized at the international, national, and state or provincial levels, Braden added. The establishment of One Health offices can foster coordination within and among these various groups and levels of organization.

Das Neves suggested leveraging political and financial power to contribute to the success of One Health agendas. In the past, individuals resisting the One Health approach have claimed that it demands a large investment with an uncertain deliverable. This argument has lost its credibility, said Das Neves. The COVID-19 pandemic has demonstrated that no matter how uncertain the deliverable of a One Health program is, the cost of inaction is far too high to put off investment, Das Neves further remarked. He expressed hope that this lesson will be applied as the pandemic subsides. In addition to international efforts from agencies such as WHO and FAO, organizing action can happen at the domestic level in the areas of education and business. Das Neves called for a coordinated, joint strategy extending beyond the connection of social science, economic sciences, and health science to perform at the local and national levels. This includes educating the private sector on the One Health strategy. Once the pandemic has been stabilized, the focus on One Health may decrease as international actors turn to address other challenges. This prospect highlights the importance of local actions, Das Neves emphasized.

Romanelli highlighted several components she considers to be essential to One Health strategies. Political will and coordinated action are instrumental for engaging all levels of governance, from local to global. At the global level, WHO provides strategic vision and oversight, but the front lines of natural resource management are at the local level. Local leaders, such as spiritual leaders and traditional medicine practitioners, should be actively engaged because they are trusted within their communities. In addition to education, developing a common narrative and vision can connect all sectors across levels of governance. Even with integrated approaches, however, new silos can be created due to the absence of a common narrative and vision, said Romanelli.

Balbus emphasized the importance of political will and leadership. Beyond merely supporting One Health, leaders must articulate its importance to bring about change in practice, Balbus said. He underscored the role of incentives within federal systems. Global health programs tend to have large budgets, which can disincentivize collaboration with other partners if agencies are wary of potentially relinquishing some of their control over overall budgets. Building in financial incentives to encourage collaboration will warrant considering the overall financial structure of systems and the flows of money within and across them. Lastly, he discussed the demonstration of value added by One Health approaches. The public health, medical, and biomedicine industries are data oriented, such that dialogues with these sectors can be framed with data to avoid giving rise to skepticism that can thwart potential collaboration. For instance, stakeholders in these industries may be skeptical of the effectiveness of interventions that focus on wildlife, ecosystems, and land management rather than on drugs or vaccines. Those working to advance the One Health approach can increase its appeal by building metrics and evaluation methods that demonstrate added value, as well as providing examples of successful One Health efforts. Balbus highlighted the need for more demonstrations of One Health approaches dealing with complex manipulations of the environment and the protection of health, such as urban wildlife interfaces, environmental chemicals and toxins, and the genetic modification of mosquitoes. Romanelli echoed the observation that the public health sector is data oriented, adding that a wealth of data is not being effectively disseminated due to gaps in cross-discipline communication (see Box 4-1). She urged advocates of the One Health approach to leverage this body of evidence in a coordinated way.

Fostering Local Efforts with Global Collaboration

Nkengasong noted that One Health programs are often highly localized in design and implementation. He asked how global policy can preserve the targeted approach while fostering necessary international cooperation. Braden remarked that animal health, human health, and ecological health are local, and interventions that work at the local level should be preserved and developed. However, developing local programs is insufficient:

BOX 4-1
Data to Support the One Health Approach

- Pandemic prevention is far less costly than pandemic response.
- Essential species are going extinct at over 1,000 times the natural rate.
- Humans have transformed three-quarters of land-based environments and two-thirds of marine environments, particularly environments not managed by indigenous communities.
- More than one-third of land surfaces and nearly three-quarters of freshwater resources are now devoted to crop and livestock production.
- More than 60 percent of infectious diseases have zoonotic origins.
- The productivity of nearly one-quarter of global land surfaces has been reduced by land degradation.
- The size of urban areas has more than doubled in the past 30 years.
- Air pollution kills over 7 million people annually.
- Subsidies and perverse economic incentives have driven dysfunctional global food and energy systems and climate change, which are expected to cause 250,000 deaths per year.
- Unhealthy diets are responsible for 11 million premature adult deaths each year.
- Approximately one-quarter of the global burden of disease is attributable to preventable environmental factors.

SOURCE: Romanelli presentation, February 24, 2021.

coordination is still needed at the state, regional, national, and international levels to affect how private-sector businesses operate. Beyond regulation, higher-level partnerships are valuable in engaging with private-sector actors. Although the private sector is ultimately motivated by financial profitability, common ground can often be found among policy makers and the private sector.

Das Neves stated that local relevance is foundational for One Health approaches; however, these cannot be duplicated from one setting to another. A greater degree of interconnection and information sharing would increase the impact of local-level solutions. For example, if one government is conducting effective surveillance in the bat population for emerging diseases, but a neighboring city 10 kilometers away is not performing any, then it reduces the overall effectiveness of bat surveillance efforts in the area. He suggested that a regional approach may be both impactful and feasible, citing the Africa Centres for Disease Control and Prevention (CDC) as an exemplar that was developed to centralize and coordinate activities within the African region. By working transnationally, regional organizations can ensure that individual, local programs are compatible with one another and that data and experiences are shared across local settings.

Romanelli emphasized the importance of connecting local, regional, national, and global efforts. United messaging and the creation of common narratives and shared vision can aid this process. As context is always a factor, solutions will need to be tailored to local settings. Moreover, sharing valuable experiences can benefit others in reaching common goals. She likened this understanding to that of the Sustainable Development Goals. It is widely understood that these will not be implemented at the local level with uniformity, yet they serve as a set of shared goals that all nations are striving to achieve. Romanelli added that working across the spheres of policy making helps to ensure alignment and coherence of policy at all levels.

Balbus pointed out that NIEHS has been building its citizen science and community-engaged research efforts for many years; they may provide helpful models for connecting local and global action.[16] These types of research can support local groups in collecting data, developing research agendas, and creating sustained partnerships. They can also serve as a powerful mechanism for connecting local efforts to broader regional, federal, and international infrastructure and funding. He noted that NIEHS has a collaborating center with WHO and 20 years of experience with sustained partnerships between core centers and community groups. These relationships have had powerful results, reflecting another way in which capacity building and equity can be incorporated into science research and public health work.

---

[16] One example that Balbus cited is the Belmont Forum. More information can be found at https://www.belmontforum.org/about/#About (accessed May 30, 2021).

Session Wrap-Up

In closing, Nkengasong invited the panelists to offer a single word that encapsulates the ideas shared during the discussion. Balbus selected "mainstreaming," noting that this is the combination of integration and coordination. Das Neves chose "commitment." Romanelli highlighted "collaborative leadership." Braden stated that "integration and mainstreaming" are integral to the concept of One Health and the progress that needs be achieved at all levels, in all sectors, and across all disciplines.

5

Building the Future One Health Workforce

This session's two plenary presentations focused on effectively training and educating the next generation of One Health professionals. Lonnie King, dean emeritus of the College of Veterinary Medicine at Ohio State University, reviewed progress in building a One Health workforce, detailed the required competencies, and outlined educational shifts needed to develop these competencies. He identified gaps in the workforce and recommended transformative changes to address them. Woutrina Smith, professor and associate director of the One Health Institute at the University of California, Davis (UC Davis), detailed current experiential-learning initiatives in Africa and Asia and described opportunities for collaboration and innovation. The session was moderated by Eva Harris, professor of infectious diseases and director of the Center for Global Public Health at the University of California, Berkeley.

THE ONE HEALTH WORKFORCE: RECONCILING COMPETENCIES WITH OPPORTUNITIES

Lonnie King, The Ohio State University

King reviewed the current status, required competencies, and anticipated future needs of the One Health workforce, with the following objectives: (1) review recent progress in building the workforce, (2) explore the most pressing needs remaining in education and the gaps in linking these needs with practical field applications, and (3) recommend transformative changes to address these issues that can be accomplished now. King quoted

Admiral Thad Allen: "Leadership is the ability to reconcile opportunity and competency" (Allen, 2010). He added that reconciling opportunities and challenges with competency is essential for an effective workforce.

Progress in Building a One Health Workforce

Currently, 45 academic programs grant One Health degrees in the United States, the majority of which have been established over the last decade (Togami et al., 2018). King remarked that global advances are even more robust, with progress in defining an effective workforce and essential competencies being demonstrated in work conducted by the U.S. Agency for International Development (USAID) in its RESPOND and PREDICT projects, the U.S. Centers for Disease Control and Prevention, the World Health Organization (WHO), the World Organisation for Animal Health (OIE) with the "Day 1 Competencies" recommendations (OIE, 2012), and One Health Institute at UC Davis with the "One Health Workforce—Next Generation" project.[1,2]

King noted that the number of scientific papers on the One Health workforce, meetings and online trainings, and assessments measuring results via tools such as the OIE Performance of Veterinary Services and the WHO Joint External Evaluation have all increased. He added that social sciences are also becoming engaged in One Health initiatives.

One Health Workforce Competencies

King remarked that "competencies" and "skills" are not interchangeable terms. A competency is an observable capability that integrates knowledge, skills, values, and attitudes. It is the "how" in effective performance. Competencies can be categorized as core, advanced, or sub-, all of which span a continuum from beginning to proficiency. In contrast, a skill is a specific ability that—when applied to a specific setting—leads to a predetermined result. In essence, it is the "what" in performance, and it may lead to proficiencies. Skills are often categorized as technical or interpersonal ("soft" skills). Investigation is under way to better operationalize and measure competency to create milestones through which students can progress across their professional curriculum, said King. A continuum of professional skills and core competencies includes the stages of novice, advanced beginner, competent, and proficient.

---

[1] The One Health Workforce—Next Generation project is funded by USAID. More information can be found here: https://ohi.vetmed.ucdavis.edu/programs-projects/one-health-workforce-next-generation (accessed May 31, 2021).

[2] King also acknowledged work performed in One Health offices across many agencies and international organizations that are not individually listed here.

In analyzing and evaluating papers written on One Health, King generated a list of key knowledge areas for the workforce. These include epidemiology, risk assessment, ecology of disease, preventive medicine, infection prevention, zoonoses, emerging infections, environmental health, health determinants, wildlife and conservation medicine, informatics, public health, surveillance, outbreaks and spillovers, global health, and understanding the dynamics at the interface of the One Health domains. King culled skill sets specified in papers and background materials to identify core competencies in an effective One Health workforce: communications, the ability to form and work in teams, systems thinking, and the ability to collaborate. Other critical skill sets include leadership at all levels; situation analysis; risk assessment; risk analysis; analytical capabilities, especially with large datasets; interpersonal skills; emotional intelligence; cultural awareness; and conflict resolution. King added that One Health employers also value problem solving, project management (being able to design a research study and take it to conclusion), stakeholder engagement, leadership ability, and change management.

Building a One Health Workforce in a Complex World

A focus on competencies is evident in a revolutionary shift in education toward competency-based curriculum that is currently taking place in the fields of medicine and veterinary medicine, said King. In the past, experts developed a curriculum and then retrofitted it to meet needs. In contrast, King noted, a competency-based curriculum begins with the needs of society and health systems, then maps these needs to the critical competencies required to meet them. At that point, a curriculum is developed to build those competencies, with attention given to the most effective ways to impart knowledge and skills. King remarked that this method of of crafting curricula starting with an environmental analysis—performed within the context of globalization, speed, and connectivity—is starkly different from traditional methods. One Health is a holistic and integrated approach, but attempts are often made to try to retrofit it into vertically oriented, siloed systems. Drawing on a term coined by the U.S. Army War College, King noted that the "VUCA" world—an environment that is volatile, uncertain, complex, and ambiguous—presents challenges to soldiers and One Health workers alike. In the current global setting, competency requires the ability to address uncertainties. King stated that "wicked problems" are those that cannot be adequately dealt with by old interventions; they require redesigned strategies or new solutions. He remarked that in a world that is rapidly changing in terms of economics, trade, health, and immigration, it can seem as if no one is in charge. Preparing a workforce with the competencies to handle this complex effort requires a paradigm shift. Independence has traditionally been common across a large number of medical sciences, but a shift toward interconnectedness is needed, King posited. Interdependence (people's mutual dependence and reliance on one another) is at the heart of the One Health approach.

Understanding and building the skills needed in a complex environment warrants a reexamination of the pedagogy, said King. Pedagogy is the method and practice of teaching and the means of imparting knowledge and skills to learners. A traditional format of a teacher-centric lecture series does not lend itself to building a One Health workforce, he remarked. A more effective pedagogy might involve experiential work carried out in transdisciplinary teams and settings, an approach that is being used in global health summer institutes. This approach lends itself to the exploration of relevant topics via case studies of antimicrobial resistance (AMR) or emerging infectious diseases, for example. A nurturing, collaborative network can also be created through these activities. Twinning programs are another form of effective pedagogy, in which faculty, staff, and students engage in a long-term immersion experience. Programs of study should be competency based, learner centered, and flexible, said King. Furthermore, interprofessional practice and education (IPE) can contribute to increasing capacity. This model has existed for half a century but has grown substantially in the last two decades. As part of a national strategy, IPE features 16–20 health science groups working collaboratively to learn and develop together while improving health outcomes in individuals and populations. Currently, 140 national centers are connected with IPE and have core competencies and goals similar to those defined in One Health. King explained that One Health is working in parallel with IPE pedagogy, offering the opportunity to combine forces to strategically improve capacity in both areas.

Workforce Gaps and Future Work Skills

King outlined current gaps in the One Health workforce. Scalability is needed to substantially enlarge the workforce at a faster rate. Training and education across life sciences can be expanded. The concept and workforce should be strongly embedded into the national security agenda and in efforts addressing health equity, he stated. Strategic involvement in these areas can foster new possibilities, understandings, partners, and resources for One Health. Additionally, key competencies and basic knowledge can be imparted to the lay workforce in order to increase understanding of and ways to use One Health professionals. Awareness of One Health concepts and utility can be expanded to other professions, employers, and the public. King suggested implementing the aforementioned pedagogical methods, with efforts to shift the focus of education from knowledge to applications. Lastly, new and relevant competencies and sub-competencies can be identified and imparted to the developing workforce to better address the challenges of the future.

King highlighted a set of driving forces identified by the Institute for the Future (IFTF)[3] as impacting the skills necessary for the future workforce, many of which are relevant to future One Health work skills. These drivers, and the associated relevant skills, include the following:

- Artificial intelligence, requiring sense-making and adaptive thinking;
- New media ecology, requiring social intelligence and new media literacy;
- Globally connected world, requiring transdisciplinary and "T-shaped" workers (those with a deep understanding of one field and the capacity to converse in a broader range of disciplines);
- Supersized social organizations, requiring cross-cultural competency, virtual collaboration, and a design mindset; and
- Computational world, requiring computational thinking, cognitive load management, and predictive modeling.

King remarked that these skills are applicable to the One Health workforce. He added that IFTF suggests that as many as one-third of currently required skills will change within the next 5 years. If this premise holds true, it implies that key skills for the One Health workforce are likely to shift as well. A skill that may become particularly relevant is the ability to use information technology for learning and for applications mastering large, disparate data flows to solve problems and gain new insights. Increasing proficiency will involve responding to unexpected, persuasive communication strategies and new media, design thinking, translating large databases, and discriminating and filtering necessary information from the noise of the system, and being a "T-shaped" worker, said King.

Big Solutions for Big Problems

King suggested that Rosabeth Moss Kanter's textbook, *Think Outside the Building*, uses an appropriate metaphor for addressing complex, intractable problems for which adequate solutions have not yet been developed (Kanter, 2020). For such issues, individuals can move beyond the confines of their "buildings" to form cross-sector coalitions that use systems thinking to generate innovative ideas and strategies. King also suggested that innovation for low- and middle-income countries can lead to substantial breakthroughs. One Health involves working across professions,

---

[3] More information about the Institute for the Future can be found at https://www.iftf.org/home (accessed on April 16, 2021).

institutions, organizations, and disciplines. Holistic dialogues can help connect the academic, medical, and agricultural silos by building collaborative, non-hierarchical relationships across sectors. The professionals in these relationships—whom King referred to as "tightrope walkers" traveling between silos—can become effective teams. He noted that this collaborative work is in progress and will continue.

King attributed a quote to Rahm Emanuel (2020), "Never waste a good crisis." The current COVID-19 pandemic is a global event that could cause losses upward of $14 trillion. An event of this magnitude requires new approaches that include consideration of actions previously deemed impossible, King remarked, and this is not the time for fundamental, incremental thinking; the current moment calls for transformative thinking and for preparing a workforce of the future that is able to take aggressive action. The World Bank has estimated that the total annual cost of building and operating One Health systems for effective disease control in all low- and middle-income countries would be $1.9–$3.4 billion (World Bank Group, 2018). King remarked that in the midst of the costly pandemic, this figure seems a bargain. He continued that the workforce of tomorrow must be built without looking backward. Harvard's meta-leadership model emphasizes the ability to lead where one does not have authority, across organizations and the private sector (Marcus et al., 2006). King called relationship building the "skill for the decade," which is pertinent within the One Health community, between health sciences, and especially in forming a new relationship of understanding and working with natural systems.

Actions That Can Be Taken Today

King presented four areas of potential actions that could build the future workforce that effective One Health practice requires. The first area is education transformation. This involves moving toward the competency-based curriculum, a step that King highlighted as critical. Increasing online global certificate programs can build capacity, and adjusting standards and accreditation encourages change. The pedagogical options discussed earlier, including IPE, are the mechanisms by which a One Health–embedded curriculum can be effectively delivered. Lastly, increased public awareness of One Health can strengthen education transformation.

In the area of relationship building, King remarked that IPE can serve as the missing link needed to build positive working relationships and collaborative networks. Relationship building can facilitate integration of strategies being brought forth by planetary health and convergence science. Rather than reinforcing silos, professionals should collaborate to combine these strategies into one cohesive future strategy—with AMR as a fulcrum—that links with health systems to sustain and protect natural systems, said King. The next action area is upskilling. This involves meta-leadership, leading across organizations and agencies without the authority to do so. The "T-shaped" experts play a role in generating upskilling capacity. Furthermore, cultural awareness is needed to build teams with diverse ideas and backgrounds. King said that the need for innovation, implementation strategies, and project management leadership cannot be overemphasized in countering a volatile, uncertain, complex, and ambiguous world.

Capacity is the fourth action area. To address many employers' unfamiliarity with the One Health workforce, he suggested creating new positions for advanced One Health experts that are specific to today's needs, such as national preparedness and response officers, specialists in reducing risks at the human–animal–environmental interface, resilience resource experts, and pandemic prevention officers. The need for One Health workers in agriculture cannot be overstated, said King. The competencies to address crop issues and infectious disease in animals are aligned with One Health workforce competencies and can be the next extension of the concept. He also recommended creating national centers of foresight, prediction, and preparation.

King asserted that the greatest barrier to systematizing One Health is trying to reconcile technological changes, economic and global integration, and emerging health threats with traditional political structures, institutional arrangements, and habitual ways of doing things. He noted that it would be unwise to formalize structures within a system that is not receptive to One Health. In designing and preparing the One Health workforce, establishing and enabling a knowledgeable One Health workplace must also be attended to, said King.

UNIVERSITY NETWORKS ON THE FRONT LINES FOR COMMUNITY ENGAGEMENT AND ONE HEALTH INNOVATION

Woutrina Smith, University of California, Davis

Smith discussed general methods of collaboration and encouraging innovation, then outlined specific activities carried out in Africa and Asia through the One Health Workforce—Next Generation (OHW-NG) project, which partners with Africa One Health University Network (AFROHUN; formerly known as One Health Central and Eastern Africa) and the Southeast Asia One Health University Network (SEAOHUN).

Practices and Possibilities

Smith noted although the current global focus is on coronavirus disease 2019 (COVID-19), another future outbreak is inevitable—it could be a different coronavirus, Ebolavirus, an arbovirus, or the like. To highlight current endeavors and possibilities in contending with the ongoing threat of outbreaks, she posed a series of scenarios and asked participants to consider whether the situations described are currently taking place or are not yet happening. The first scenario was being a phone call or e-mail away from communicating with colleagues on every continent. Smith stated this is currently taking place, and that efforts should continue in building a global network of health professionals committed to a One Health approach. Next, she presented the scenario of students regularly attending class with students based in other countries. This is not happening often. However, just as this workshop featured speakers from around the world connecting, such classes are a possibility that could become reality. Smith suggested that regularly bringing students together worldwide would help foster global citizenship and enable students to thrive. Furthermore, students could be encouraged to innovate and to share ideas via competitions for innovation. She remarked that holding innovation competitions provides a local context for applying and adapting ideas to make them effective. Students are the future, and the field can help them become leaders and systems thinkers through application-based competitions. Team-based problem solving being the norm was the next scenario. Smith argued that it is not yet the norm but is an achievable goal, with momentum building in that direction. She posited that teams collaborating across sectors and disciplines will be most effective in finding sustainable solutions. Finally, Smith introduced a scenario in which finding and working with colleagues from government, academia, and the private sector is easy. Despite challenges involved in realizing this scenario, ideas are being generated to overcome them, which is an important step toward implementing this best practice.

COVID-19 is a tragic wake-up call, and we need to be ready for the next pandemic, said Smith. Stories of resilience and innovation have emerged, and professionals are working to capture lessons learned to prepare for the future. The One Health approach considers connections among humans, animals, plants, and their shared environments in generating integrated solutions. She remarked that this will not be the last pandemic, so the One Health approach will be invaluable in moving forward effectively together as a global community during the next crisis.

One Health Workforce—Next Generation

Smith highlighted USAID's contributions, including the Emerging Pandemic Threats program and PREDICT, which focused on surveillance and on-the-job training, and the One Health Workforce project. Currently, the OHW-NG project, an $85 million training arm funded for 2019–2024, focuses on pre-service education and experiential learning. A global team works with AFROHUN and SEAOHUN at international, regional, and local levels. The goal of OHW-NG is to empower One Health university networks to sustainably develop and deliver world-leading model programs for equipping professionals with transdisciplinary skills to address complex global health issues. Smith noted that this involves creating space to innovate and providing networks with frameworks for adaptation and success into the future.

The OHW-NG project supports SEAOHUN, AFROHUN, and member universities in workforce empowerment, knowledge management, organizational sustainability, and gender issues. Workforce empowerment involves developing and delivering trainings in alignment with prioritized One Health core competencies and technical skills. Smith noted that in this effort, OHW-NG is working to decolonize global health. This living experiment involves shifting project leadership from primarily being based in the United States to the regional One Health university networks over the 5-year span of the project. This includes much twinning and operationalizing of business practices. Knowledge management includes establishing systems and strategies to evaluate performance and track workforce placements. Organizational sustainability is achieved by strengthening the capacities of regional One Health university networks for direct donor funding acquisition and management. The project supports gender integration as a core competency and includes gender considerations as a crosscutting theme. The training in the One Health approach is critical to the program, said Smith. She highlighted the need to empower local leadership to strengthen capacities in the long term, as some U.S.-based funders and organizations may not remain in the system indefinitely.

Training the Next Generation of One Health Leaders

Smith stated that SEAOHUN is operating in eight countries with 87 member universities and ministries and 28 One Health student clubs. Operating in nine countries with 18 member universities and 16 student One Health clubs, AFROHUN is expanding and developing a greater presence in West Africa, fostering collaborations, and recruiting faculty and students for many different types of training. Highlighting the recent work by student groups, Smith presented a video featuring a student reporting on Uganda's Students One Health Innovations Club response to the COVID-19 pandemic (see Box 5-1). Smith remarked that these students are active, highly motivated, and serving on the front lines in their communities. As the pandemic developed, OHW-NG was working to build a global One Health community of practice. Many countries across Africa, Asia, Europe, and North America participated in interactive online sessions. The student role in local-level work and in community engagement has been critical, Smith noted.

> **BOX 5-1**
> **Uganda Students One Health Innovations Club**
>
> As the global community raced to slow the spread of COVID-19, the Uganda Students One Health Innovations Club (SOHIC) joined the global fight. It organized a response with two objectives: (1) raise awareness about accurate COVID-19 information and (2) support implementing public health interventions as guided by the Uganda National Health Task Force and WHO. Once a national state of emergency was declared in Uganda, over 20 One Health students in Mbarara volunteered in Mbarara Regional Referral Hospital to support the COVID-19 task force. The SOHIC at Mbarara University of Science and Technology responded by organizing an online webinar, which trained several international students from Uganda, Kenya, India, and other countries. They organized a needs assessment to assess gaps in knowledge, attitudes, and perceptions about COVID-19. The gaps were used to influence and inform a community information dissemination program that answered community questions and displayed posters about COVID-19 in both English and Luganda. Ninshaba Jacob, a student involved in the effort, said, "There's no point of me going home to protect myself. This is the kind of work I choose and the kind of life I'm going to live for the rest of my years."
>
> SOURCE: Smith presentation, February 24, 2021.

Echoing King's earlier presentation, Smith stated that competent One Health practice "is not just about what you know, it's what you know how to do." Using the competency approach, OHW-NG is developing an AFROHUN and SEAOHUN One Health Workforce Academy that will become live in 2021. She highlighted One Health innovations that are already taking place in Africa and Southeast Asia in areas including robotics, reducing exposure and contact in health care settings, and developing innovation and training approaches at the local community level. Virtual platforms and e-learning are used to both connect students across many countries in classroom instruction and create field-based experiential learning opportunities. Student One Health clubs are an avenue for delivering hands-on training; over the past year, this has taken place on the frontlines of the pandemic response, with students leading COVID-19 risk communication and community-engagement campaigns. Using the One Health approach, students conduct needs assessments and raise awareness about COVID-19 and other health issues. Smith noted that this is an active area of work, and OHW-NG plans to continue updating methods, incorporating innovations, and strengthening partnerships with local organizations and ministries of health, all of which foster sustainability of this One Health innovation project. Partnerships involve fellowships and internships, in which students gain real-world experience working with COVID-19 response teams. Mentoring activities include students and faculty collaborating to create COVID-19 awareness videos, posters, and flyers. Smith shared that One Health digital awareness challenges have fueled these activities. A student competitor reflected on the experience: "We learned to be open minded to the opinion of others, to collaborate with each other. We also learned a lot about COVID-19 and how to influence others through online platforms." Smith remarked that it is not possible to train everyone to be experts, but it is feasible to train people to be observant and use their experiences to come up with locally relevant solutions.

Another initiative, One Health Champions, was created to foster leadership and acknowledge innovation. Smith noted that many annual reports and publications feature practitioners' successes, such as faculty members who recognize and promote the value of the approach and students demonstrating leadership in One Health clubs. Smith added that some One Health Champions work in Rwanda, a nation that has long committed to a One Health approach from the top down; this provides students with new opportunities for surveillance and training.

In spite of limitations created by COVID-19, in the past year OHW-NG has trained 22,569 individuals, mentored 46 student clubs, and conducted 51 activities increasing capacity to respond to the pandemic. The project has reach and plans to achieve scalability in applying best practices to new areas, said Smith. One Health puts technical knowledge and innovation into a social context—with crosscutting themes of economics and culture—that can elucidate how myriad diverse aspects of an issue relate to one another and inform the development of effective solutions, Smith emphasized.

DISCUSSION

The Role of Citizen Science in One Health

Harris asked whether citizen science might play a role in priming students of today to become good One Health agents of public health in the future. Additionally, she queried how the existing resources of pooled data and an interested public might be leveraged to strengthen the One Health approach. King remarked that the current moment provides an opportunity to engage stakeholders and the public to be more involved in One Health. He elaborated that citizen science does not merely provide researchers with valuable yet inexpensive data; it can improve a society's broader involvement in, engagement with, and understanding of issues related to One Health efforts. Smith added that citizen science approaches are becoming more common, noting that the observational powers of the public can be helpful, with experiential learning offering an avenue for engaging the public and helping them understand that they are part of the solution.

Overcoming Funding Shortages

A workshop participant noted that while academia and public education have valuable roles to play in building a future One Health workforce, schools and universities are struggling to pay for existing programming during the current funding crisis. The participant asked how One Health advocates might navigate the potential lack of receptiveness to new initiatives that educational institutions may have at this juncture. Smith acknowledged that the funding challenges are real, yet One Health can be part of the solution. As an example, she suggested that it can assist with building a diversified business model for finding innovative methods to access funding sources. She remarked that public–private partnerships can be explored for added value and collaboration beyond the public and academic spheres. In the OHW-NG project, specific private-sector partners are coming forward and offering support, such as fellowships for intern placements. Whenever possible, these types of relationships should be encouraged to broaden the inclusivity of One Health efforts, said Smith. King commented that the COVID-19 pandemic has demonstrated how video meetings can help to build capacity, because they enable collaboration without requiring participants to convene in one physical location. He added that Smith is using video meetings in OHW-NG activities, proving that capacity building does not necessarily require significant increases in funding to merit results. Exemplifying this, a program was recently hosted by Cornell University's College of Veterinary Medicine, a local health system, and the New York department of public health, which trained 1,000 people with One Health competencies to address COVID-19.[4] While this activity was carried out quickly and relatively inexpensively, it effectively develops beginning-level expertise, said King.

Increasing Public Trust in Scientific Experts

Another participant asked how to address the general public's skepticism or unwillingness to listen to expert advice on infectious diseases. King remarked that the current polarization of the United States has had an

---

[4] This series of online training courses for the New York State Public Health Corps drew on the Master of Public Health program in the College of Veterinary Medicine at Cornell University and collaborated with Northwell Health System. More information can be found at https://news.cornell.edu/stories/2021/01/cornell-help-train-states-pioneering-public-health-corps (accessed May 31, 2021).

impact on many individuals' beliefs in science, resulting in trust deficiency. He stated that forcing ideas on people who are not ready to receive them only adds to polarization. Instead, time should be spent expanding the groups that do believe in expert scientific advice. Additionally, the speaker delivering a message affects receptivity, said King. Smith added that while this dynamic may be more apparent in the United States currently than in previous times, it is not a new phenomenon. For instance, some people have doubted the existence of Ebola for many years. Locally credible and knowledgeable individuals with access to communities can be effective in sharing messages in digestible ways. Students and faculty have made progress in effectively engaging with community leaders and groups, said Smith. People will not change behaviors unless they believe in the need to do so, and the One Health approach places technical knowledge into social contexts in digestible ways.

Grade-School Education Efforts

Harris asked about the role that primary and secondary school education might play in One Health's sustainability efforts. Noting a comment that Kent Kester, vice president and head of translational science and biomarkers at Sanofi Pasteur and moderator of an earlier workshop session, made about the potential to spread One Health messaging through schoolchildren as has effectively been done in the past with education efforts on recycling, King remarked that grade-school education can be a useful strategy. Children in elementary and middle schools are captive audiences that often take in messaging and then share it with their parents. In this way, grade-school students can become a collective force for changing habits and behaviors. Smith stated that similar efforts are taking place in the food safety and infectious disease sectors, where children in the United States and other countries are taught in the classroom and given homework assignments that bring those lessons into their home environments. For instance, they may be asked to count the eggs their chickens produce or be tasked with keeping a notebook of chickens' disease symptoms. Such real-life applications can help children understand these concepts at an early age; this understanding can then become internalized by the time they grow into adulthood. Smith suggested that "working upstream" in this way can be effective.

One Health Certificate

A participant asked if a One Health degree program would offer an advanced degree geared toward upper management positions or if it would be a professional certification designed for early career individuals and students. Noting the concept of the "T-shaped" professional, Smith stated that professionals must have expertise in one area and a general awareness of the importance of collaboration and interdisciplinary work to have a role within a One Health team. Thus, a One Health certificate serving as an advanced credential might be most effective. Such a certificate would not replace One Health awareness efforts at earlier stages of education; rather, it would serve as an additional layer to be earned by professionals. A certificate would indicate soft skills that are valued by One Health employers, such as integrating ideas, working well on a team, and using systems thinking. King added that One Health degree programs are also attractive in early careers. Furthermore, employers need to become knowledgeable about the benefits these competencies bring to the organization. He remarked that building skills and knowledge is a lifelong pursuit of continual improvement, as it is with leadership skills.

Addressing Opportunity Inequality in Health Care

Harris asked about the role that One Health can play in deracializing, decolonizing, and improving equity in health care professions, given the lack of diversity in high-level health care careers in the United States and the financial and opportunity barriers to attaining such positions. Smith replied that this important question does not have clear answers but suggested expanding the current methods of extending One Health opportunities in knowledge, experience, and collaboration. Successes in these efforts can be used to establish best practices moving forward. Currently, veterinary schools in the United States are building on efforts made in the human health sector to increase diversity in incoming cohorts of students. Health professionals are beginning to consider needed steps in this area, but this work is in early stages, said Smith. King added that One Health emphasizes prevention and early detection. Approximately one billion people in the world's lowest-income countries depend on plant and animal agriculture, so efforts to prevent infectious diseases and bolster nutrition are critical to achieving health equity. One Health focuses on preventing infections, which can have a profound impact within populations that are more likely to be severely infected by infectious diseases.

Role of Modeling Expertise in Expanding Prediction Capability

A participant stated that improving predictive capabilities and prevention at the source involves engaging infectious disease and landscape ecologists and mathematical modelers to merge complicated methodologies. The participant asked whether One Health education efforts include these disciplines to strengthen prediction and prevention. Smith replied that in her work on the PREDICT project, on-the-job training approaches were used with country-level teams in collecting data, applying it to predictive models, and using the predictions to improve readiness moving forward. As OHW-NG is a training arm, the program routinely carries out this work. However, expansion of efforts in this area is needed to reach university and in-service audiences, said Smith. Foundational knowledge must be established before highly sophisticated methods can be learned, creating a spectrum of learners at various stages and levels of competency. Smith suggested that projects should continue to focus on increasing these capabilities.

King remarked that over the past 5 years, impressive advances in data analytics have resulted in new resources and opportunities for exploring datasets such that data analytics has become an additional area of proficiency for One Health professionals. He added that increasing focus on foresight and protection—by creating three national centers on foresight, prediction, and preparedness—is a feasible step toward optimizing the use of data analytics.

Environmental Justice and One Health

Harris asked the panelists for suggestions about how to incorporate conversations about environmental justice into One Health education. Smith noted that in the classes she teaches, students have some choice in the topics they address, and environmental justice issues are becoming more popular. Initially, this area was not a central One Health focus, she explained. However, One Health is a responsive, collaborative approach in which faculty and students learn from one another, so professionals should give this area of increasing demand more attention. King emphasized that One Health should first define societal needs and problem areas, then design competencies and curricula based on those needs. Interest is increasing in environmental science, environmental health, and equity, so One Health should incorporate this area into its purview, said King.

Preventing the Siloing of One Health Education

A participant noted that the aim of One Health is to combine disciplines, but the Western education system is likely to relegate it to a single specialty within a discipline rather than take a more holistic, cross-disciplinary approach. The participant asked if the One Health education's ability to achieve its ultimate integrative goal necessitates changes in the overall way science is taught. King noted a Massachusetts Institute of Technology paper that identified three major transformation areas in science: molecular biology, genomics, and convergence science (Sharp et al., 2016). Convergence science brings together disciplines to create new opportunities, and the National Science Foundation has allocated $30 million to growing convergence research as one of the organization's "10 Big Ideas" for pioneering research and pilot activities.[5] This focus on convergence science is an opportunity for One Health to avoid a singular disciplinary approach, said King. Smith added that One Health is an approach, not a discipline. Rather than designing a specific course or degree program, educators can incorporate One Health as a crosscutting theme. At UC Davis, funding was invested in a multi-campus effort to build topics related to sustainability, health, and the environment into the curricula of schools of medicine, pharmacy, and nursing. This effort did not mandate new courses. Instead, specific examples of the One Health approach can be used in conveying the concepts courses already address, updating curricula to incorporate the One Health approach.

REFLECTIONS ON DAY 2

Harris highlighted key themes and concepts from the panel discussions and plenary presentation session, and Peter Daszak, president of EcoHealth Alliance and member of the planning committee, summarized the presentations heard on day 2 of the workshop. The first panel discussed long-practiced efforts that fit within the One Health model yet are only recently being referred to as One Health practices, such as research on food-borne illness that uses an interdisciplinary genetics approach and the area of plant health that can serve as a model system for human health in terms of aerial surveillance and modeling communities and populations. The role of plant health and the impact of environmental disruptions on new diseases were discussed, with emphasis placed on the need to include plant health within One Health.

Panelists discussed an understudied area in the use of systems thinking and data analytics to understand the complexity of how components of an issue fit together. During-action reviews conducted in the midst of a crisis were discussed as helpful tools that can identify new resources in surge capacity, risk evaluation capacity, and epidemiology across sectors; they can also be leveraged to develop policies and resource sharing. Harris pointed out that community-based efforts were exemplified through engaging the Maasai population in Tanzania in the design of data collection tools. Involvement of the private sector, with Harris highlighting the use of natural history collections, such as the *Outbreak: Epidemics in a Connected*

---

[5] More information about the National Science Foundation's 10 Big Ideas can be found at https://www.nsf.gov/news/special_reports/big_ideas/index.jsp (accessed April 18, 2021).

World exhibit.[6] Panelists explored the importance of breaking down silos and cautioned that even One Health programs have a risk of developing silos of animal, public, and ecosystem health.

In the second panel session, panelists focused on the need to expand One Health approaches both upward into leadership levels and downward into the workforce. Modernization of antiquated ideas and data collection systems and strategies for institutionalizing collaboration integration, including the establishment of data-sharing policies and standard operating procedures across agencies, were discussed. Additionally, the need to look at root causes and build resilience with equity was emphasized. Panelists considered the benefits of incorporating ecological and environmental dimensions and noncommunicable diseases into the One Health approach. Harris noted that the overarching themes of this panel discussion were mainstreaming, commitment, collaborative leadership, and integration.

King and Smith spoke on the competencies, skills, and milestones; the concept of competency-based education and curriculum; experiential pedagogy; and interprofessional education and practices that can build the future workforce. King pointed out that gaps in scalability, expansion across education sectors, embedding key competencies, and shifting knowledge to application exist in the current workforce. Addressing these gaps will require de-siloing, transformative thinking, relationship building, upskilling, and capacity building. The discussion addressed the role of citizen science, primary- and secondary-school education as an avenue for One Health awareness, becoming a "T-shaped" professional with both expertise and cross-disciplinary knowledge and competency, using One Health to decolonize and deracialize education and the workforce, and the concept of convergence science. Harris noted the emphasis on One Health being an approach, rather than a discipline.

Daszak expanded on Harris's reflections by highlighting the theme of connectivity in the panel discussions and presentations. This connectivity is between people, livestock, and wildlife, and the current framework of rapid socioeconomic and environmental changes fuels a breakdown of interactions between them. He noted that some countries are making greater progress than others in using One Health as a central planning strategy for major health threats, such as emerging diseases, and that this progress has often been made in the context of experiencing repeat issues in recent years. The need for prominent use of a One Health approach in all countries and at all levels, from local to global, has emerged as a theme in this workshop, he added. Daszak described the COVID-19 pandemic as a One Health

---

[6] A digital version of the exhibit was created in response to the COVID-19 restrictions and can be found at https://naturalhistory.si.edu/exhibits/outbreak-epidemics-connected-world (accessed May 31, 2021).

issue, because the virus spread through the interface of people, livestock, wildlife, and the environment. A more structured One Health approach may enable outbreaks to be stopped early on or even prevented entirely; one that is applied in every country and supported by global cooperation and collaboration could prevent some critical issues, such as pandemics, Daszak suggested.

6

Learning from the Past and Planning for the Future of One Health

The third session focused on innovative technologies, frameworks, and collaborations that could mitigate future pandemic threats. The session's objectives were to discuss (1) lessons that can be learned and extrapolated from the coronavirus disease 2019 (COVID-19) pandemic, including priority actions for policy, public–private partnerships, and industry resilience to build a broad, threat-agnostic global health system and (2) strategies to facilitate international cooperation and data sharing to establish forecasting capabilities for emerging health threats. Jonathan Quick, managing director of pandemic response, preparedness, and prevention at The Rockefeller Foundation, discussed possible detection and response mechanisms of the future that would enable outbreaks to be swiftly controlled before becoming pandemics. Katherine Huebner, veterinary medical officer at the U.S. Food and Drug Administration's (FDA's) Center for Veterinary Medicine (CVM), and Danielle Sholly, animal scientist at FDA CVM, discussed the threat of African swine fever (ASF) and its global impact. They outlined features of the One Health approach FDA uses in addressing this infectious disease. John Amuasi, co-chair of the Lancet One Health Commission and leader of the Global Health and Infectious Diseases Research Group, Kumasi Centre for Collaborative Research-Kwame Nkrumah University of Science and Technology, Ghana, highlighted the role of prevention policy, the paradoxical nature of resistance to prevention efforts, and the impacts of health inequalities and prevention inequities on individuals and nations simultaneously facing poverty and viral outbreaks. Rajeev Venkayya, president of the global vaccine business unit at Takeda Pharmaceutical Company Ltd. and member of the board for Coalition for Epidemic Preparedness Innovations (CEPI), reviewed advances in vaccine innovation during the COVID-19 pandemic. He outlined preclinical, clinical, and manufacturing measures that could accelerate the development of vaccines for novel viruses. The session was moderated by Peter Daszak, president at EcoHealth Alliance.

PRECISION EPIDEMIOLOGY, HUMAN BEHAVIOR, AND THE FUTURE OF ONE HEALTH

Jonathan Quick, The Rockefeller Foundation

Imagining future possibilities in outbreak detection and response, Quick described a scenario in 2035 in which an outbreak is swiftly controlled and ended within 100 days. He suggested possible advances in collaboration, methodology, and technology that would enable this vision to become reality. Quick discussed current efforts to improve the data pathway to increase the speed with which infectious diseases can be detected and controlled. Highlighting that goals deemed impossible may actually be feasible, he provided examples of progress made in outbreak response over the past 50 years.

The 2035 Pandemic That Wasn't

Quick remarked that the next generation will inherit advances and challenges from the generations before it. Imagining the future they will inhabit, he painted a scenario illustrating the continuum of animal and human health and what might be expected in the year 2035. In this scenario, ongoing, routine zoonotic surveillance is performed. Big data are used, including human data, microbial or health service data, data related to climate change, and animal and vector data. Artificial intelligence fuels geo-risk assessments used to determine priority surveillance locations. Point-of-contact surveillance is performed in communities. Risk-based assessments inform onsite, viral genomic surveillance in animals, and routine surveillance takes place in humans and animals that are particularly at risk.

The scenario then forwards to 30 days before the imagined outbreak. At this point in the future, much has been learned about key genes and about how genes in animals may affect humans. Some patterns emerge in 2035 that are associated with virus transmission to humans, based on genomic sequencing. When a worrisome virus is spotted, more intensive animal sequencing is performed to look for patterns associated with deadly virus strains. More intensive surveillance of humans also commences, particularly on those in contact with at-risk animals.

Fast-forwarding to 15 days before the outbreak in the scenario, the alert level is increasing. Targeted testing and screening are increased to a wider geographic area. The hypothetical Global Genomics Surveillance Center is alerted, and the center notifies national authorities and local human and animal services to increase vigilance.

A large portion of the population owns wearable electronic devices, as inexpensive models are widely available, and device privacy is fully protected. On day 0 of the outbreak—when the first case is reported—individuals receive health alerts on their devices. The "astute clinician"[1] is aware of the alerts and suspects a novel virus. Genome sequencing confirms a new, previously unknown virus strain. On day 1, the frontline sequence is deposited in a global viral sequence repository, where it is made available to governments, universities, and industry worldwide. Diagnostic and therapeutic professionals assess what steps may be necessary for humans and animals, and vaccine development begins.

By day 7, airborne transmission is confirmed, making the virus highly transmissible among humans. The first virus-attributed deaths take place, and some cases require extended hospitalization. In the year 2035, 3-D printing of diagnostic tests is feasible, and tests become available now. Local actions are set into motion, including social distancing, masks, quarantining, and the at-home "lollipop" testing developed through technology advancements. Global travel alerts are sent to the general public, and targeted, big-data travel patterns are performed. High-risk arrival locations conduct point-of-entry screening for that genome.

At day 60, therapeutics have already been developed and vaccines are becoming available. A variety of methods provide accelerated safety and efficacy testing far faster than in 2021. Advancements in manufacturing enable rapidly deploying vaccines in accordance with hot spot vaccination plans. Vaccines are even produced in patch form, making needles and syringes unnecessary; these are manufactured on 3-D printers and delivered via drones, increasing scalability. All other expected public health measures are in place.

On day 100, the last case is reported. Shortly thereafter, the outbreak is declared over.

Strengthening the Data Pathway for Outbreak Detection and Response

Quick stated that "the die is cast" during the first 100 days of an outbreak. Even the first few days of response to the initial case substantially affect the speed of exponential growth of an infectious disease. Thus,

---

[1] Quick noted the "astute clinician" term applies to practitioners such as Carlo Urbani, the first person to identify severe acute respiratory syndrome (SARS) as a new virus, and Zunyou Wu, who was among the first scientists to study severe acute respiratory syndrome coronavirus 2 (SARS-CoV-2), the virus that causes COVID-19.

actions taken in the early days can result in many lives saved. However, containing outbreaks requires informed, targeted action by a range of actors, and current systems to detect and respond to outbreaks are weak (see Figure 6-1). To strengthen systems, Quick shared, the Rockefeller Foundation is researching how big data can inform the action platform and rapid response. This involves examining the timetable of an outbreak, identifying critical actions and responses, and determining how to build the data needed to initiate those actions. Steps of the data pathway from source to user could include (1) collecting diverse data inputs; (2) aggregating, coordinating, synthesizing, and sharing data; and (3) leveraging data to drive action. Strengthening this pathway involves generating robust data inputs, harvesting data, making data publicly available in real time, finding ways to navigate governmental efforts to limit data sharing, and incorporating novel sensors, Quick pointed out. Examples of novel sensors include frontline workers in health, veterinary medicine, or forestry services who are able to log test results with a smartphone. Advanced big data management and artificial intelligence are combined with scenario planning to generate action plans.

Quick described a vision for what this hypothetical world-class pandemic action and data sharing platform could yield:

> We envision a global platform that will become a leading force for amplifying warning signals and containing the spread of pandemic-potential outbreaks within their first 100 days—delivering the best information to the actors positioned to take action that averts the most devastating human and economic impacts of pandemics.

The health, social, and economic effects of pandemics interrelate. Quick noted that pandemics lead to three categories of deaths: (1) caused directly by the virus, (2) related to a disruption of health services, and (3) connected to economic disruptions. Providing an example of the third category, Quick stated that in the 2008 Great Recession, cancer deaths in Europe and North America increased by 250,000 due to impacts caused by economic disruptions.

Imagining the Impossible

Quick remarked that much about the 2035 scenario he described may seem impossible at this moment. Urging the audience to "imagine the impossible and then make it happen," he provided three examples of revolutionary global health efforts. The first was smallpox, which Europe and North America eradicated by 1950, Quick pointed out. In 1953, George Brock Chisholm, the first Director-General of the World Health Organization

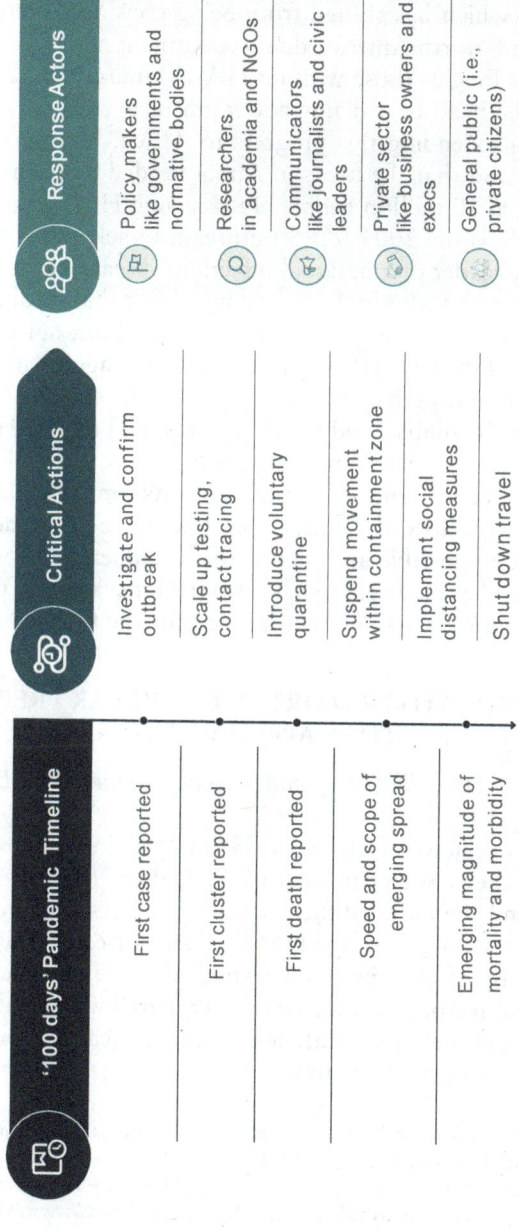

FIGURE 6-1 Critical actions and response actors involved in outbreak containment.
NOTE: NGO = nongovernmental organization.
SOURCE: Quick presentation, February 25, 2021.

(WHO), proposed global smallpox eradication (Bhattacharya, 2008). However, the World Health Assembly did not vote to do so until 1966. Quick noted that some decision makers thought this was impossible, yet it was accomplished in 1980. Another example is the human immunodeficiency virus (HIV), which has shifted from being considered terminal to chronic in Europe and North America due to treatment advances, with people living almost as long as those without HIV (Marcus et al., 2020). Quick said that when the head of a major development agency was asked about the possibility of extending this progress to Africa, he responded that it was not possible and that the focus in Africa needed to remain on prevention. A decade later, 10 million people are receiving HIV treatment in Africa. A third example is the 2003 SARS outbreak. Quick stated that in March of that year, the leader of a national infectious disease agency was questioned about eliminating SARS by June, and he replied that he did not think it was feasible, but the outbreak was over by July and has not returned.[2]

In terms of the COVID-19 pandemic, 1 year ago, many experts thought that by this point, perhaps three or four vaccines with 50 percent efficacy rates might be available, said Quick. However, at the time of the workshop, eight vaccines are in late stages of approval, most of which are more than 70 percent effective, and more than 200 million doses have been administered in 99 countries.[3] Quick noted that in each of these cases, people imagined the impossible and then made it happen. He concluded that it is possible to make the world much safer from devastating global pandemics if people commit to making their visions for the future a reality.

COLLABORATIVE EFFORT IN OUTBREAK PREPAREDNESS: FDA'S APPROACH TO ASF

Danielle Sholly and Katherine Huebner, FDA

Huebner reviewed features of ASF and its global impact. She discussed the roles of the U.S. Department of Agriculture (USDA) and FDA in containing it, and she outlined the activities of FDA's ASF work group. Sholly discussed key strategies of the FDA ASF Draft Response Plan. Highlighting the complexity of effectively addressing ASF, she provided an overview of the One Health Approach for Disease Preparedness collaborative response framework and the appropriateness of a One Health approach for meeting the threat of infectious diseases.

---

[2] More information about the 2003 SARS outbreak is available at https://www.cdc.gov/sars/about/fs-sars.html (accessed May 27, 2021).

[3] The numbers cited by Quick were accurate as of February 2021. For more updated status of vaccine development, approval, and distribution, see https://www.who.int/publications/m/item/draft-landscape-of-covid-19-candidate-vaccines (accessed July 7, 2021).

ASF

A highly contagious viral disease, African swine fever (ASF) results in hemorrhagic fever of both domestic and wild pigs.[4] Huebner noted that while ASF spreads rapidly and has high morbidity and mortality rates, it does not affect the health of animals other than swine and is not transmissible to humans. It has never been detected in the United States; if it were introduced, it would have devastating economic impacts for the nation, said Huebner. Disease transmission is influenced by human, animal, and environmental factors. Given that the virus can persist stably in the U.S. environment, it can be transmitted through contaminated materials, such as livestock transport trucks. Feeding pigs uncooked food waste ("swill") and contaminated meat or carcasses can also result in transmission. An active area of research is the viral transmission of ASF through contaminated manufacturing of animal feeds, spreading the virus via feed mill equipment and the feed itself. Viral vectors include flies, soft ticks, and wildlife reservoirs, such as warthogs and wild boars. No vaccine or treatment is available, although developing novel vaccines is an active area of research. Challenges to these efforts include insufficient knowledge of protection mechanisms and of the antigens involved in this large, complex ASF virus. The primary methods of virus control are preventative biosecurity measures and the depopulation of affected or exposed swine.

Huebner stated that ASF has caused significant pig losses globally. Endemic to sub-Saharan Africa, the disease emerged in Eastern Asia in August 2018, where it expanded uncontrollably and resulted in substantial losses. According to a 2020 World Organisation for Animal Health (OIE) report, Asia suffered the greatest impact, with more than 6 million animals lost (OIE, 2020). This accounts for at least 80 percent of the total global losses reported to date. During this period, several countries in Eastern Europe reported the first cases of ASF, which were followed by uncontrolled spread and devastating impacts. While ASF is not a direct threat to human health or human food safety, it is a major threat to animal health and global food security, Huebner explained. For example, mass animal depopulation and subsequent animal disposal present major animal welfare and environmental safety challenges, in addition to the economic impact on farmers and communities who must depopulate their animals. Animal losses also affect the availability of safe sources of protein for human and animal consumption. Modeling predicts that the ASF-related decline in Chinese pork production will result in world pork prices increasing by 17–85 percent (Mason-D'Croz et al., 2020). In addition, unmet

---

[4] More information about ASF is available at https://www.aphis.usda.gov/aphis/ourfocus/animalhealth/animal-disease-information/swine-disease-information/african-swine-fever/seminar (accessed February 4, 2022).

demands for pork products have translated into price increases for beef and poultry, she noted. Supply chain disruptions can occur for downstream materials derived from pig tissues, such as animal feed and pharmaceutical products, including replacement heart valves and insulin. Given the variety of interconnected impacts of ASF, the multidisciplinary, multisectoral, and multilateral One Health approach—and adequately allocating resources to implement it—are key in controlling further spread and preventing its introduction to the United States, said Huebner.

The U.S. Governmental Response to ASF

As ASF has not yet been detected in the United States, the U.S. government has emphasized prevention, detection, and response planning, Huebner stated. Typically, USDA serves as the lead agency in prevention and surveillance efforts for foreign animal disease prevention. FDA's focus is the review and approval of potential viral mitigants that meet the definition of a food additive or animal drug. Charged with ensuring a safe animal feed supply, FDA is responsible for all domestic and imported animal food, with the exception of meat, poultry, and processed eggs, all of which primarily fall under the USDA Food Safety and Inspection Service. FDA monitors and sets standards for livestock feed and pet food contaminants, approves safe food additives for animal use, and manages a medicated feed program. Under the Swine Health Protection Act,[5] USDA is responsible for regulating food waste—such as garbage—that may contain meat products and is fed to swine to ensure it is properly treated to kill disease organisms. Under the Food Safety Modernization Act Preventive Controls for Animal Food Regulation,[6] FDA is involved in preventing food safety hazards of food for all animal species and applies primarily to non-farm facilities.

The FDA ASF work group was formed in 2019 to coordinate a disease response plan promoting outbreak preparedness, said Huebner. The group collaborates with USDA, state regulators, and the animal food industry. Additionally, the work group coordinates with FDA's China Office to establish joint USDA–FDA inspections in Chinese pet food facilities. Comprising representatives from USDA, FDA, the pork and animal food industries, and academia, the Feed Risk Task Force shares ideas and discusses the latest ongoing research. In addition, FDA produces a field bulletin, which alerts staff conducting foreign inspections of appropriate biosecurity measures to

---

[5] Swine Health Protection Act, Public Law 96-468, § 2, (October 17, 1980), 94, 2229.

[6] More information about the Food Safety Modernization Act Preventive Controls for Animal Food regulation can be found at https://www.fda.gov/food/food-safety-modernization-act-fsma/fsma-final-rule-preventive-controls-animal-food (accessed April 20, 2021).

take when performing inspections in ASF-positive regions. A major focus of the work group has been developing the FDA ASF Draft Response Plan, Huebner noted.

FDA's ASF Draft Response

Sholly remarked that the draft response plan created by the FDA ASF work group has been reviewed by FDA and USDA, and final comments are currently being addressed. The group used incident command principles to manage an FDA ASF response. The plan has two main objectives: (1) identify critical activities to detect, respond to, and contain ASF and prevent further spread of the disease in animal food and (2) facilitate swift normalization and distribution of animal food in affected areas. The plan addresses FDA authorities, roles, and resources needed to respond to an ASF outbreak, which is an example of the chain of command and unity of command principles that are part of the incident command program. Sholly explained that this principle clarifies reporting relationships, eliminates confusion, and provides incident managers with a framework for controlling the actions of personnel under their supervision.

The draft response plan contains three key strategies, Sholly outlined. The first is maintaining the ability to provide clean animal food, thus protecting animal health. This involves economic trade in ensuring that products imported into the United States are ASF free. Second, given that ASF can spread from an infected location, such as a farm or feed mill, the plan outlines biosecurity measures for investigators to address during inspections. These measures extend beyond the facility itself to include assessing clothing, vehicles, and equipment, as these are all possible avenues for virus transmission. The plan's third strategy is to conduct "trace forward" and "trace back" investigations on contaminated animal food or ingredients, which can involve collecting records on those distributed by a particular facility. Sholly noted that in an ASF outbreak, the ability to identify contaminated animal food or ingredients in a timely manner decreases the likelihood that distribution of non-contaminated animal food to animal production facilities and farms in surrounding areas will be disrupted.

In addition to the draft response plan, the FDA ASF work group is involved in public outreach efforts, said Sholly. These include an ASF webpage[7] on FDA's CVM website that provides a high-level overview of ASF with links to information resources and offers transparency on the center's response to this foreign animal disease. She noted that the webpage states CVM's commitment to working with sponsors to facilitate the

---

[7] The FDA ASF webpage can be found at https://www.fda.gov/animal-veterinary/safety-health/african-swine-fever (accessed April 20, 2021).

review and approval of products intended to prevent ASF infection and viral spread.

Collaborative Response Framework

Highlighting the importance of a One Health approach in disease outbreak preparation efforts, Sholly described the complexity of a highly contagious virus such as ASF. In the scenario of a group of feral pigs being infected with ASF, a "stamping-out strategy" from USDA's drafted *African Swine Fever Response Plan: The Red Book*[8] begins with depopulating the animals. The next step of the coordinated response is designating zones around the site where the infected pigs were located. The immediate area around the site is designated the "infected zone," and a broader ring is a "buffer zone," which is surrounded by a third, larger "surveillance zone." These zones are used to inform quarantine and movement control efforts, which may involve multiple agencies from the federal, state, and local levels. Sholly emphasized that features of the location or feral swine population, such as population density and proximity to county or state lines, can increase the complexity of the response efforts exponentially.

In spite of the various resources informing prevention and containment efforts, ASF remains a deadly disease, said Sholly. Cross-sector collaboration to prepare for an outbreak includes tabletop exercises in which representatives from USDA, FDA, and the swine industry work together to develop and review response steps. These exercises familiarize representatives with the reasoning behind each of the plan's action steps. Representatives identify the parties responsible for carrying out the activities, proactively preparing them with necessary tools to provide a rapid response to an incident. FDA and CVM are working with USDA and state regulators to expand upon existing collaborative efforts in managing an outbreak response. Sholly remarked that disease outbreak preparedness reveals the value of enhanced communication and coordination among different stakeholders.

The Role of One Health in Effective Response

The intersection of human, animal, and environmental health is evident in the efforts required for effective disease outbreak preparedness, Sholly stated. Therefore, FDA uses a One Health approach in addressing the threat of ASF. This includes collaborating with other stakeholders, identifying anticipated challenges specific to ASF, using risk mitigation, considering

---

[8] The USDA *African Swine Fever Response Plan: The Red Book* is in draft form and can be found at https://www.aphis.usda.gov/animal_health/emergency_management/downloads/asf-responseplan.pdf (accessed April 20, 2021).

all potential routes of viral transmission, safely transporting animals and food, and taking biosecurity measures. FDA highly values the ongoing enhancement of collaboration and coordination with other government agencies and industry entities, said Sholly. She continued that although collaborating to implement a One Health approach is not always easy, it increases the likelihood of achieving the best possible outcomes. Much has been learned from past and present human and animal disease outbreaks, such as COVID-19, bovine spongiform encephalopathy (commonly referred to as "mad cow disease"), and porcine epidemic diarrhea. FDA and CVM remain committed to protecting the safety of humans, animals, animal food, and the environment in the face of disease threats and outbreaks, Sholly remarked. The success of any response plan relies on following the science and working as a team to expeditiously resolve an outbreak. Sholly closed with a quote from President Dwight Eisenhower, "In preparing for battle I've always found that plans are useless, but planning is indispensable."

PARADOX OF GLOBAL POLICIES FOR PANDEMIC PREDICTION AND PREVENTION

John Amuasi, Global Health and Infectious Diseases Research Group Kumasi Centre for Collaborative Research—Kwame Nkrumah University of Science and Technology, Ghana

Amuasi described the increase of national and individual challenges at the intersection of viral pandemic and poverty. He outlined the theory of fundamental causes of health inequalities and the "prevention paradox," discussed in detail later. Highlighting the role of prediction and prevention policy, Amuasi described the resistance that the prevention paradox can instill in the public and in decision makers. He emphasized the equity issues at play in prevention efforts and called for greater international cross-sector collaboration to create a healthier world.

Intersectionality of Poverty and Pandemic

Amuasi stated that One Health has become particularly topical during the COVID-19 pandemic.[9] The burdens of epidemics and pandemics are evident on the global economy, medical health systems, social systems, and general development (WHO, 2018). He noted concerns that COVID-19 may necessitate backtracking in development plans for West

---

[9] Amuasi referred the audience to the "Policies, Politics, and Pandemics" June 2020 issue of the International Monetary Fund bulletin, *Finance and Development*, found at https://www.imf.org/external/pubs/ft/fandd/2020/06/pdf/fd0620.pdf (accessed April 20, 2021).

African countries that were still recovering from the Ebola epidemic of 2014 to 2016, such as Guinea, Sierra Leone, and Liberia. As controlling Ebola required these countries to become familiar with various containment measures, they were able to implement COVID-19 mitigation strategies fairly quickly. However, the "double whammy" of COVID-19 and poverty-related diseases increases the burden for low-income countries, Amuasi described. Guinea is currently experiencing another Ebola outbreak and just recently began vaccination efforts, so it must navigate simultaneous COVID-19 and Ebola vaccination campaigns.

All health crises disproportionately affect the poor due to the impacts of limited availability, accessibility, and affordability of health services and the disruption of existing programs aimed at addressing that lack of services, said Amuasi. When zoonotic disease is layered with poverty, the "double whammy effect" can be both direct and indirect. The severity and mortality of COVID-19 are strongly associated with nutritional status and age. Various neglected tropical diseases and infectious diseases associated with poverty cause immunosuppression, which can increase vulnerability to COVID-19 and other epidemic- and pandemic-prone diseases. Therefore, an individual living in poverty with an underlying health condition and poor nutrition is more prone to a severe or mortal case of COVID-19, experiencing a "direct double whammy," Amuasi remarked. He elaborated that indirect ramifications of this intersection of poverty and pandemic include disruptions of (1) routine services, such as mass drug administration for helminthiasis, a parasitic worm infection; (2) the manufacturing of drugs, diagnostics, and vaccines for diseases other than the pandemic; and (3) health service delivery activities, such as surgeries for buruli ulcer, lymphatic filariasis, and trachoma.

The Prevention Paradox

Geoffrey Rose described a "prevention paradox" that occurs when population-based prevention health measures—such as compulsory seatbelt laws, alcohol taxes, and mass immunization—bring large benefits to a community but may offer little benefit to nonparticipating individuals (Rose, 1985), Amuasi explained. Rose proposed placing a greater focus on shifting the entire population into a lower-risk category than on moving high-risk individuals into normal range. Given that a large proportion of the population is at moderate risk before intervention, efforts to move this group to low risk contributes to the greatest overall benefit. Amuasi pointed out that several actions made in the public interest during the COVID-19 pandemic have been met with resistance, even from some people who ordinarily make well-informed decisions. He suggested that to comprehend such paradoxes around policies aimed at predicting and preventing pandemics, one must first understand the nature of health inequalities. Global forces, political priorities, and societal values create fundamental causes of unequal distributions of power, money, and resources (Link and Phelan, 1995). Distribution disparities affect wider environmental influences and, in turn, individual experiences in the areas of economics and employment, education, services, and social, cultural, and physical experiences (Beeston et al., 2014). Inequalities in these wider influences and individual experiences lead to inequalities in the distribution of health and well-being.

The absolute version of the prevention paradox occurs when consensus is achieved by individuals who do not want to participate in a policy measure addressing a population-level concern, said Amuasi. They prefer no population-wide preventive health strategy, viewing their individual benefit as very low and dismissing considerations about the benefit for the overall population (Thompson, 2018). He noted that the protests in the United States, Europe, Asia, and Africa against lockdowns intended to mitigate the spread of COVID-19 are examples of this paradox (Holligan, 2021; Wilson, 2020). Individuals who do not expect to experience personal gain from population-based preventive health measures may prefer not to be subjected to them.

Prediction and Prevention Policy

This prevention paradox can affect pandemic response mass vaccination efforts, said Amuasi. The challenge in working toward COVID-19 herd immunity when a percentage of the population resists being vaccinated underscores the utility of One Health approaches. He stated that pandemic prediction and prevention require integrated animal and human surveillance systems in wildlife, domesticated animals, livestock, animals in cities, and humans in urban and rural areas (Amuasi et al., 2020a). These areas interact in complex ways, and multiple conditions likely contributed to the cross-species transmission of COVID-19—including to humans. Therefore, global policies are needed at all levels of epidemic efforts, Amuasi emphasized. Effective management begins with prediction and detection early in an outbreak (WHO, 2018). Once transmission is detected, containment measures are instituted. As the outbreak amplifies, control and mitigation measures can reduce transmission until the virus is eliminated or eradicated. The policies needed to conduct these multi-level epidemic management efforts are inherently complex. Amuasi highlighted a report from the Intergovernmental Science-Policy Platform on Biodiversity and Ecosystem Services (IPBES) that details the relationship between biodiversity and pandemics and proposes cogent solutions (Daszak et al., 2020).

In advocating for prediction and prevention policies, some claims are safe to make, as they have been proven to be accurate, while others require more information (Aberdeenshire Community Planning Partnership and What Works Scotland, 2018). For example, it is clear that many prevention efforts are cost effective, said Amuasi. Using an "upstream" approach, prevention policies often address the fundamental causes of health inequalities before problems arise, increasing the quality of human life and proving to be cost effective. However, prevention will not necessarily result in cost savings. Amuasi noted a differentiation in the terms "cost-effectiveness" and "cost savings." Additionally, while evidence supports a shift to prevention, precisely pinpointing efforts that are most cost effective is not possible, he stated.

Paradoxical Challenges to Prevention Efforts

Amuasi shared that his team is conducting seroprevalence field studies in Kumasi and Accra, two cities in Ghana. These studies involve both interviews and blood sample collection. Currently, these efforts are fairly well received due to the COVID-19 pandemic. He stated his expectation that outside a pandemic situation, routine surveillance requiring people to answer questions and provide samples would be met with considerable resistance; many people would likely not understand why they should comply. Complex questions arise, which require multidisciplinary training and involvement to address. Amuasi noted a conundrum that researchers face: the more successful prevention efforts become, the weaker the arguments for policies and investment in population-level interventions may seem. Decision makers and the general public may not intuitively understand the need to spend money on an issue that is not visible. The absence of outbreaks may suggest that the global health of the public no longer requires interventions, which can lead to the resurgence of epidemics. Another challenge in instituting global prediction and prevention policies is variance in value systems, said Amuasi, which can complicate consensus-building in terms of the subpopulations that constitute risk groups and the policies to protect them. For example, as the population in Africa is largely young, African decision makers may not view older people as a priority group, in contrast to countries such as Japan or Switzerland, he remarked. When consensus cannot be reached about the subpopulations that are at risk, it is challenging to agree on which policies to create and enact, Amuasi stated.

Prevention Equity

Amuasi emphasized that an additional challenge in effective prevention efforts is achieving equity. Issues of equity and solidarity are common, caused by access barriers to medical countermeasures, particularly for low-income countries and nations facing humanitarian emergency, he described. Access inequity increases when vaccine or treatment production is limited. Thus, global prevention policies must be fair and equitable in order to be effective worldwide. On February 24, 2021, Ghana was the first country to receive COVID-19 vaccines through COVAX, a vaccination collaboration that includes Gavi, WHO, CEPI, and the UN Children's Fund (Mawathe, 2021). Ghana received 600,000 doses of the AstraZeneca vaccine, yet its population is approximately 40 million people, said Amuasi. While Ghana will receive future shipments, the COVAX policy assures that participating countries will receive doses for only 20 percent of their populations. Thus, nations are still faced with the challenges of accessing vaccines for the majority of their residents. This demonstrates that even strong global policies may be insufficient for the comprehensive global prevention of outbreaks, Amuasi stated.

Given the prevention paradox, discrepancies in prevention efficacy emerge even within a country. Furthermore, global prevention policy can reinforce inequities; in strengthening it, policy makers must consider whether changes will benefit only select countries and continents, said Amuasi. He highlighted a recommendation in the IPBES Workshop on Biodiversity and Pandemics report:

> Launching a high-level intergovernmental council on pandemic prevention that would provide for cooperation among governments and work at the crossroads of the three Rio conventions to: 1) provide policy-relevant scientific information on the emergence of diseases, predict high-risk areas, evaluate economic impact of potential pandemics, highlight research gaps; and 2) coordinate the design of a monitoring framework, and possibly lay the groundwork for an agreement on goals and targets to be met by all partners for implementing the One Health approach (i.e., one that links human health, animal health and environmental sectors). (Daszak et al., 2020, p. 5)

Creating a high-level Intergovernmental Council on Pandemic Prevention would be a complex endeavor, but this is the type of action that is needed, he stated. In a coauthored piece in *The Lancet*, Amuasi called for establishing a COVID-19 One Health research coalition that would build on the urgency generated by the pandemic to strengthen collaboration with climate change and planetary health communities (Amuasi et al., 2020b). He remarked that the pandemic is a turning point in the history of the world, one the general international community can meet by designing, undertaking, and coordinating supplies and research aimed at promoting a healthy and sustainable planet.

TAKING PANDEMIC THREATS OFF THE TABLE

*Rajeev Venkayya, Global Vaccine Business Unit,
Takeda Pharmaceutical Company Ltd.*

Venkayya outlined progress made in outbreak threat awareness and vaccine innovation during the COVID-19 pandemic. He described the prototype pathogen strategy, which could substantially accelerate the time required to take a vaccine candidate to trial for an emerging threat. Outlining additional preclinical, clinical, and manufacturing efforts in preparing vaccine platforms in advance, Venkayya noted steps needed toward greater equity in vaccine access. He described an aspirational goal of shortening the development time for novel virus vaccines to 100 days.

Advances Made During the COVID-19 Pandemic

Venkayya stated that this is an extraordinary time in vaccinology. He commented that over decades of development and innovation, the activity over the past year has never been seen before. The COVID-19 pandemic has brought advances in threat awareness, vaccine platforms, and strategies. Worldwide, eyes have been opened to the magnitude of the threat of pandemics and the art of the possible. COVID-19 has made it clear that pandemics can be caused by viruses other than influenza, and coronaviruses have now matched influenza in terms of threat, said Venkayya. Threat awareness extends to the global community now understanding that animal populations can act as reservoirs in the future. The response to the pandemic has revealed the power of rapid sequence sharing, which continues to be called on as new variants emerge.

Advances during the COVID-19 pandemic include creating new vaccine platforms, Venkayya remarked. Messenger ribonucleic acid (mRNA) is an exciting technological development garnering much attention in the scientific community. In addition to nucleotide-based vaccines, other platforms—including vectored vaccines, subunit approaches, and novel adjuvants—have been developed. He noted that risk is associated with platforms that involve growing viruses in cell culture and taking accurate measurements from assays to determine the quality of product consistency. Given this risk, the gap between the performance of mRNA and other platforms was shorter than may be the case in future pandemics, said Venkayya. Regardless of whether that proves to be the case, a range of platforms suitable for the pandemic threat exists. The discovery of a number of new strategies can speed the time to product availability for large populations. He commented that the most important innovations have involved risk-based approaches to development, performing some actions at risk that typically would be carried out in sequence. Additionally, innovative approaches have embraced the concept of meeting the threat at its source. For example, Operation Warp Speed established clinical trial sites across the United States in an effort to rapidly demonstrate proof of efficacy in the communities being hardest hit by the pandemic.[10]

While the COVID-19 pandemic has been met with increased awareness and innovation, it has brought considerable response challenges. The risks involved in the biology of vaccine production, particularly for the non-mRNA vaccines, have emerged, said Venkayya. Inevitably, problems arise in virus growth, cell growth, consistency of the product in process testing, and quality control deviations that delay the arrival of supply. He stated it is not surprising that manufacturers of many COVID-19 vaccines have seen reductions in the expected volumes they are able to produce within a given time frame. Assays have proved challenging, in terms of both the tests used and the clinical assays evaluating immunogenicity in humans, the validation of which involves specific challenges. The complexity of the biology of traditional vaccine manufacturing and the uncertainty involved in growing viruses and cells pose challenges. Venkayya noted this as an area in which the mRNA platform has a distinct advantage.

Prototype Pathogen Strategy

The lessons learned during the COVID-19 pandemic provide an opportunity to rethink how pandemic preparedness should be approached in the future, Venkayya remarked. He stated an ultimate goal of removing pandemic threats altogether. To this end, CEPI is actively evaluating the concept of prototype pathogens, which represent the characteristics of families of viruses that could emerge as human pathogens. He noted approximately 23 current virus families. While influenza and coronavirus are likely top priorities, research can extend to other families in advance of the next pandemic. This strategy involves identifying a range of tools and even candidate vaccines for virus families, reducing the time between a specific virus emerging as a pandemic threat and candidates being developed and taken to human clinical trials.

Two years before COVID-19, Barney Graham and Nancy Sullivan outlined the exact approach that was later used to develop the first severe acute respiratory syndrome coronavirus 2 (SARS-CoV-2) vaccine candidate (Graham and Sullivan, 2018). Venkayya explained that this approach centers on rational vaccine design, which begins with understanding which epitopes are most important on the surface of the virus and for cell entry.

---

[10] More information about Operation Warp Speed is available at https://www.defense.gov/Explore/Spotlight/Coronavirus/Operation-Warp-Speed (accessed May 27, 2021).

That knowledge is converted to an understanding of the antigens or immunogens that would be most effective in generating a useful neutralizing antibody response to that pathogen. Various platforms that prove to work against the virus are then applied. Testing these in animal models in advance of an epidemic develops understanding of immune correlates of protection. Ideally, vaccine candidates can be evaluated in phase I clinical trials to assess both initial safety and immunogenicity (the generation of an antibody-mediated immune response cell that appears to correlate with a protective response in animals). The ability to carry out this strategy could enable a toolkit of vaccine candidates across multiple families and possibly including multiple candidate vaccines within a given virus family. Venkayya remarked that this could substantially accelerate the timeline to clinical trial material and the availability of vaccines against an emerging pandemic threat.

Preparing the Platforms

A range of vaccine development activities can be performed in parallel to accelerate vaccine timelines, said Venkayya. Preclinical efforts include animal models, which require time to develop and validate. Work on animal models can be performed now, he noted. Toxicity studies can be carried out on the platform itself. For example, in developing the mRNA platform, toxicity studies had been conducted on humans for multiple mRNA vaccine candidates over the past decade, which fostered understanding of toxicity before SARS-CoV-2 emerged. Reproductive and other assessments can be performed to provide further confidence in the safety of vaccine candidates before they are administered to humans in a phase I trial.

Venkayya noted that phase I trials for selected vaccine candidates could take place before a pandemic begins. Clinical trials for safety and immunogenicity need to be easy to mobilize and implement quickly, given the lack of ability to predict exact locations of outbreaks, he remarked. The ability of organizations such as WHO and CEPI to implement clinical trial protocols in an outbreak setting will increase the likelihood of collecting useful data on the vaccine candidate within a matter of weeks. Expansion is also possible in chemistry, manufacturing, and controls, a technical and complex area. The inherent challenge is bringing what works in a laboratory to a commercial scale, said Venkayya. For example, traditional, inactivated, vectored, recombinant vaccines must be manufactured in the range of hundreds or thousands of liters at a time. He remarked that mRNA vaccines have an advantage, as a chemistry-based approach like mRNA does not have the complexities that come with scaling up a viral vaccine or producing virus in a bioreactor. Regardless of whether the platform is mRNA, optimizing scale-up strategies before the threat can be valuable. Venkayya stated that it may not reduce the time for a vaccine to reach the clinic, but having evidence demonstrating that a product works can shorten the time between data collection and producing a substantial vaccine supply for the world.

Product assays, which include potency assays and other quality control assays used throughout the production process, must be validated and maintained from a quality standpoint to enable confidence in the process. Venkayya added that with vaccines, "the process is the product" due to the lack of effective methods of characterizing the complex biologic that is a traditional vaccine. He pointed out that this is not the case for mRNA. However, the limitations in accurately characterizing traditional vaccines require that a robust and reproducible process that includes appropriate quality control testing throughout be used to ensure consistency. In regard to manufacturing at scale, Venkayya highlighted that bringing new manufacturing facilities online to make products that they have never produced before is extremely complicated. It involves both infrastructure needs and reusable component needs, which are typically varied from company to company and product to product. Changing one element of the manufacturing process necessitates a bridge showing that the attributes of the product are unchanged.

Equity and Manufacturing Expansion

Addressing equity issues before the next pandemic will require increased distributed manufacturing capability and capacity, said Venkayya. An inequitable distribution of the first doses of safe and effective COVID-19 vaccine resulted in some regions of the world having early access to substantial quantities, while the vast majority of the world had little to no access. This inequity has fueled consideration of the requirements to expand self-sufficiency in vaccine manufacturing beyond Europe, the United States, and parts of Asia to countries in all regions of the world. Venkayya noted that mRNA vaccines present an opportunity in this area. The complexity of traditional vaccine manufacturing prohibits immediately establishing new manufacturing capability in a country. Developing the workforce skill, capacity, and regulatory experience required for traditional vaccine manufacturing is far more time intensive than building a factory. These surrounding ecosystem elements are important in maintaining high-quality manufacturing. In contrast, chemistry-based mRNA vaccines have greater predictability and less manufacturing complexity. He remarked that mRNA vaccines could be a gateway technology for countries that have never manufactured vaccines, enabling them to "leapfrog" more traditional methods. Venkayya emphasized that he does not suggest that mRNA vaccines will solve all problems. With current technology, mRNA vaccines are not effective for all viruses. Technology may improve to enable greater application, and at minimum, an mRNA vaccine strategy needs to be developed in preparation for the next pandemic, he said.

A Vision for Future Outbreak Response

Venkayya highlighted an aspirational concept of decreasing the timeline between sequence identification and phase III data submission and availability of vaccine supply to only 100 days.[11] With COVID-19, the time from WHO receiving genetic sequencing of the novel coronavirus to the submission of the first phase III data to regulatory authority was slightly over 300 days. Venkayya noted that this is an incredible achievement. He likened the aspiration to speed up vaccine development and shorten this time frame to only 100 days as similar to proclaiming the goal of landing on the moon; no exact plan exists to achieve this goal, but areas are being targeted for innovation that could lead to accomplishing it.

While this goal may be accomplished, it will not be possible to achieve for every pathogen, said Venkayya. For example, no effective HIV vaccine exists. Although developing vaccines for some pathogens is highly challenging, other viruses are more straightforward; for these viruses, the 100-day goal is within closer reach. The United Kingdom is pushing G7 to undertake this target, and CEPI is giving it serious consideration. Venkayya remarked that shortening the vaccine development time will serve as a North Star for CEPI post-COVID-19.

DISCUSSION

Data-Sharing Considerations

Given that improving outbreak response time relies on prediction capability—and that high-quality global data sharing is needed to advance that capability—Daszak asked how the security of data and data users can be protected while simultaneously enabling better access to data. Quick cited ongoing efforts to address the challenge of data security, which involve both technical (e.g., in terms of how data are filtered) and governance solutions. He noted that part of the solution is creating more transparency in how data sharing is overseen, which can enable protections to be built in. Quick remarked that in a pandemic, the right to privacy can interfere with the right to health and life, necessitating certain tradeoffs. Striking the appropriate balance is challenging, however. He remarked that some

---

[11] An overview of the vaccine development and regulatory approval process can be found at https://www.fda.gov/vaccines-blood-biologics/development-approval-process-cber/vaccine-development-101 (accessed July 7, 2021).

of the countries with the most effective COVID-19 responses, including Singapore and South Korea, have mostly managed to protect privacy while saving lives. Quick added that some apps were not protected and noted that ensuring data security can involve balancing conflicting rights, requiring ethical judgments to be made.

Impact of Trade Issues on Data Sharing

Daszak asked Huebner and Sholly about their approach to data sharing with China, as trade issues became a key global political issue.[12] Given that addressing ASF requires openness and access to sensitive information on swine production in China that affects global health and trade issues, Daszak asked how they approached acquiring access to data. Furthermore, he queried whether the strategy they used could be scaled up to encourage a broader initiative, such as a global health data network. Huebner replied that she works primarily with the USDA, which has the lead U.S. government role on this issue. In 2020, the United States and China engaged in a phase one trade agreement[13] that established purchasing targets for some U.S. commodities, including pork. She noted that FDA and USDA are engaged in implementing the agreement to open up exports of pet food, feed additives, premixed compound feed, and distillers grains to China. Such collaborations around trade can improve the global health network, said Huebner.

U.S. ASF Testing Capacity

A participant asked whether U.S. national and state animal laboratories have the resources needed to ramp up ASF testing. Sholly replied that this falls under USDA's jurisdiction. USDA has worked with their network of laboratories on testing and testing capacity in case ASF is ever detected in the United States. USDA's *African Swine Fever Response Plan: The Red Book* outlines sample collection and diagnostic testing and identifies the National Animal Health Laboratory Network in providing standardization and response testing for any foreign animal diseases. She added that as of April 2020, six U.S. laboratories are approved to test for ASF.

---

[12] The United States entered a trade war with China in July 2018, when plans were announced to impose tariffs on $450 billion worth of Chinese goods (Swanson, 2018).
[13] More information about the U.S.–China phase one trade agreement can be found at https://ustr.gov/phase-one (accessed April 22, 2021).

Equitable Representation in International Planning

Referencing the IPBES panel Amuasi served on, Daszak broached the idea of creating a similar One Health panel. He asked how, if created, the panel might approach ensuring that experts from low- and middle-income countries are given leadership roles. Daszak added that many successful, national-level One Health projects are carried out by low- and middle-income countries. Amuasi suggested looking beyond a panel to forming a high-level council focused on pandemic prevention. This council would reach consensus on priorities and lead countries in establishing mutually agreed-upon targets and goals within the framework of a core agreement. Amuasi reiterated that determining who is at risk, how best to address those risks, and variances in value systems are areas that can be challenging in achieving consensus. He described that to participate in the IPBES process, his request to participate had to be approved by Ghana governmental representatives. In a similar manner, experts serving on an intergovernmental council on epidemic preparedness could function as representatives of their respective countries. This would ensure representation from the Global South, which is particularly needed in addressing the issue of variance in a value system, said Amuasi. For example, while completing a questionnaire for the Lancet-Chatham House Commission, he was tasked with selecting priorities for reducing the impact of climate change. However, he felt the projected priorities were not adequately sensitive to different value systems. The challenge lies in ensuring that a variety of values are represented, he emphasized.

Balancing Vaccine Development Profitability and Access Equity

Daszak noted that Venkayya is a member of the board of CEPI, which takes a global approach to vaccine development, as well as being employed by a for-profit pharmaceutical company. The vision of a broad vaccine platform toolkit would involve companies sharing development strategies, which could put profitability at risk, Daszak pointed out, and asked how for-profit companies will be able to collaboratively share data, frameworks, and access to the ultimate product. How can profitability and access equity be balanced? Venkayya replied that CEPI is well positioned to address this challenge. Having gained experience in Lassa fever, Nipah, Middle East respiratory syndrome (MERS), chikungunya, and Rift Valley fever, CEPI is prepared to move forward with an emphasis on new pandemics. Venkayya described a scenario in which CEPI supports multiple companies and platforms, allocating targets or possibly even vaccine constructs for different companies to put on their platforms. Notably, CEPI would fund this work. As for-profit companies must generate return and continue to fund innovation, they are unlikely to invest research and development funds into developing a vaccine for a hypothetical threat. Thus, CEPI funding for this work is important, said Venkayya. The concept of governments supporting this type of research and development through an entity such as CEPI is a new innovation, he added. As research and development are highly complex, most governments are not comfortable making those investments. CEPI can play a valuable role in funneling government investments into allocations across companies, Venkayya noted. Furthermore, he posited that companies will feel confident receiving constructs from CEPI, knowing that these constructs have gone through some level of vetting. In this scenario, companies will not have to determine which vaccine construct to use; rather, they will be given the construct and then apply their platform to it.

Valuable Skill Sets in One Health

A student participant earning a master of public health degree asked which skill sets are most needed in the next generation of public health professionals and epidemiologists. Daszak asked the speakers to identify some skills that will enable operationalization of a forward-thinking strategy; the predictive, global, and collaborative vaccine platform; and One Health on-the-ground approaches. Quick replied that a wide variety of skill sets can have an impact, so a student's particular talents will inform the areas that will be of most benefit to pursue. He added that during the pandemic, the tactical use of videoconferencing has proliferated, but the collaborative benefit of this technology has yet to be optimized. He likened this to a child who knows the mechanics of picking up a phone and talking on it but does not understand the social aspects of how to carry on a phone conversation. Quick said that effective use of videoconferencing will expand collaboration and open possibilities in every area.

Venkayya responded that the pandemic has highlighted the value of contributions from a broad range of backgrounds in developing an effective response. He noted that data science and real-world evidence are two priority areas moving forward. Tightly controlled clinical trials have long been considered the primary means of gathering data, and evolution is needed to further expand data collection efforts, said Venkayya. Data system development in advance of an outbreak will enable early data collection. He remarked that situational awareness with high-fidelity data would be incredibly valuable.

Amuasi studied in both Ghana and the United States, and he earned a minor in development studies and social change. He stated that this education was valuable in shifting his perspective on how the world works and how scientific research should be performed. His work has ranged from understanding snake bites in rural Africa to conducting clinical trials and seroprevalence studies for COVID-19. Amuasi suggested that students pursue an understanding of the complexity of the world, which includes awareness of what one does not know. Understanding one's knowledge gaps enables a person to seek out team members with the expertise to fill those gaps. Daszak added that expertise in unusual side issues that may not seem critical can become valuable within a multidisciplinary team. This adds diversity, and all forms of diversity bring value, said Daszak.

Advancing a Proactive Response in a Political Climate

Daszak noted that when a novel disease outbreak occurs, a global response requires governments' willingness to implement drastic response measures. This took place in China early in the COVID-19 outbreak, but perhaps it might have been possible to put Wuhan on lockdown 1–2 weeks earlier, he surmised. Given the natural tendency to underreact in order to avoid political fallout for instituting severe restrictive measures, Daszak asked about strategies to implement a predictive framework more proactively. Sholly replied that this is a challenging issue requiring tough discussions. Establishing open communication and collaborations before an outbreak can enable prompt interagency discussions once an outbreak occurs. As each agency has individual expertise in a specific area, familiarity with the network of agencies makes it possible to contact the appropriate experts when a need related to a projected disease is identified. She added that this can include state and local entities as well. For example, if an ASF outbreak occurred, swine producers, packing facilities, rendering entities, and veterinarians would need to be made aware. Sholly noted that the tabletop exercises are beneficial in raising awareness of the complexity and severity of the issue for stakeholders. Huebner acknowledged the sensitive nature of this topic, given the trade-off in the benefit of alerting the industry and various stakeholders early on versus the harm that can result with fallout to the response. It can also be difficult to determine the level of threat. For example, a prominent issue surrounding ASF testing and laboratory results is whether a positive test indicates live virus or a fragment of dead virus; for the latter, it is unclear whether this signifies that ASF has been introduced to a new region, said Huebner.

Quick remarked that this is a "damned if you do, damned if you don't" scenario. He recalled that when an outbreak of swine flu occurred in 1976, the director of the U.S. Centers for Disease Control and Prevention called for mass immunization; however, when the virus did not go global, the director was fired.[14] He stated that WHO overreacted to the H1N1 outbreak in

---

[14] More information about the 1976 Swine Flu vaccination program is available from https://wwwnc.cdc.gov/eid/article/12/1/05-1007_article (accessed April 30, 2021).

2009, declaring it a pandemic and later rescinding that declaration, and that this fueled the organization's reluctance to declare COVID-19 a pandemic.[15] Quick identified three areas for improvement in addressing this tension between underreaction and overreaction. First, better decision tools are needed. While much attention is given to modeling virus behavior, modeling efforts on human behavior are inadequate. Better decision tools could make responses more specific and appropriate to the threat. Second, awareness efforts can better prepare the public, stakeholders, and business community over time. Third, annual rehearsals allow practice during a calm state; rehearsals can increase the likelihood of appropriate decision making during an emergency. Quick noted that when cabinet responsibilities are transferred in the U.S. government, incoming cabinet secretaries are informed about pandemic response, but this can get lost in the delivery of copious information.

Shifting to a Preparation Mindset for Disease X

Daszak noted the difficulty in past years of mobilizing even a fraction of the billions of dollars spent on the COVID-19 response—a disease that has cost trillions of dollars in losses—toward Disease X preparedness.[16] He added that "Disease X" is a misunderstood term, as some people erroneously believe that COVID-19 is Disease X, and therefore it is no longer necessary to prepare for it. Daszak asked how to shift the reactive psychology and instill the understanding in governments and taxpayers that funding Disease X preparedness can save billions of dollars and potentially millions of lives. Venkayya stated that pandemic preparedness is about imagination. He described that during his involvement in U.S. government work on pandemic preparedness, discussions of community mitigation strategies such as closing schools were met with resistance. However, the COVID-19 lockdowns extended far beyond what he and his colleagues envisioned. While lockdowns are not the solution to all pandemic-related issues, this example illustrates that in the face of a threat, people will do what is necessary to save lives, said Venkayya. The global trauma caused by the pandemic has stretched the collective imagination. Furthermore, as deadly as COVID-19 has been, it is possible that a Disease X could be even worse. Viruses have been detected with higher lethality or higher transmissibility, so a future novel virus could potentially lead to a worse pandemic than the current one.

---

[15] More information about the declaration of the COVID-19 pandemic is available from https://www.chathamhouse.org/2020/05/coronavirus-public-health-emergency-or-pandemic-does-timing-matter (accessed April 30, 2021).

[16] "Disease X" was used in the WHO priority diseases list as a placeholder for "a serious international epidemic" that is currently yet unknown and may occur. For more information, see https://www.who.int/activities/prioritizing-diseases-for-research-and-development-in-emergency-contexts (accessed July 7, 2021).

Venkayya emphasized that while the threat of a future pandemic is present in public awareness, an opportunity exists to access resources needed to launch a preparedness initiative. His ultimate goal is to remove the threat of pandemics altogether. New tools have proven to be effective, and experts are able to map out the requirements to reduce the time to vaccine availability and substantial supply. CEPI is actively working toward implementing this road map. The U.S. Biomedical Advanced Research and Development Authority (BARDA) continues to work in the space as well. In addition, the European Union is developing the European Health Emergency Preparedness and Response Authority, which will serve in a similar capacity to BARDA. Furthermore, the African Union is involved in efforts to speed vaccine development. Venkayya stated that this is the first time in history that tools are in place to be able to mitigate a pandemic threat; sustaining momentum could drive substantial change.

Amuasi reflected on the role of the past Ebola outbreak in preparing Africa to contend with COVID-19. He noted that Ebola is more deadly than COVID-19 and that its presence in Africa required systems and capacities to be put in place. Without these response efforts to Ebola, the challenges COVID-19 posed in Africa would likely have been even greater, said Amuasi. The pandemic serves as "the great reset," an opportunity to do things differently. Newly implemented systems enable advances in research on drugs, vaccines, diagnostics, and the clinical characterization of unknown diseases. Amuasi leads the operational readiness and response work package for the African coaLition for Epidemic Research, Response, and Training (ALERRT), a consortium of 19 partner organizations from 13 African and European countries. ALERRT has instituted measures that allow research to begin as quickly as possible when an epidemic or pandemic occurs anywhere in Africa. These efforts proved successful in addressing outbreaks of monkeypox and plague, and ALERRT is currently active for Ebola, indicating that prevention and response mechanisms can be effective. By instituting these mechanisms fairly early during the COVID-19 pandemic, Africa was able to mitigate the impact. However, funding is needed to capitalize on scientific advances. He remarked that funding allotted toward some of the negative externalities of the pandemic is more than twice that for the fundamental causes. Amuasi continued that left unaddressed, these fundamental causes will continue to put humans at risk of yet another Disease X, a threat that never disappears completely and is ever-present.

7

Building a Better System for Outbreak Response, Surveillance, Detection, and Forecasting

In-depth breakout discussions were held to discuss key, feasible goals and steps that can be taken toward improving outbreak preparedness efforts for the future. Organized by topic, breakout groups included response capacities, surveillance and detection mechanisms, and forecasting and predictive innovation. Each group was tasked with identifying short-term goals, long-term goals, and potential actions and relevant institutions involved in achieving these goals. Jonna Mazet, professor and founding executive director of the One Health Institute at University of California, Davis (UC Davis), moderated the breakout room recaps and discussion.

BREAKOUT SESSION HIGHLIGHTS

Response Capacities

Kent Kester, vice president and head of translational science and biomarkers at Sanofi Pasteur, moderated the breakout discussion focused response capacities (see Box 7-1). He highlighted short-term goals identified by participants, including addressing areas of improvement that emerged in the coronavirus disease 2019 (COVID-19) pandemic response. Notably, personnel development is needed in professional, governmental, and nonprofit sectors, as well as at the community level, summarized Kester. This involves training for the entire continuum of One Health human resources. Furthermore, an inventory of human resources in the current One Health workforce can aid in identifying gaps and ensuring that all health providers are included. He pointed to insufficient data regarding international spending

> **BOX 7-1**
> **Highlights from Discussion on Response Capacities**
>
> *Presented by Kent Kester, Sanofi Pasteur*
>
> Short-term goals:
> - Evaluating human resources in the current One Health workforce and ensuring that all health providers are included.
> - International Monetary Fund monitoring spending on public health capacities to address the lack of data.
> - Integrating risk communication into the One Health approach.
> - Integrating the agriculture sector into the One Health approach.
> - Engaging citizen scientists and bolstering community-level surveillance.
>
> Long-term goals:
> - Improving health literacy.
> - Broadening engagement in One Health to include the arts, literature, broad social sciences, communication skills, cultural awareness, and humility.
> - Building capacity to measure improvement.
>
> Immediate feasible actions:
> - Improving training in One Health for all health care providers from the ground up.
> - Expanding data collection to include spending that strengthens public health capacities; monitoring data collection to ensure that it is sustained during non-crisis periods.
> - Bringing other sectors to the table in One Health, particularly experts in social science, anthropology, psychology, and agriculture.
> - Leveraging opinion leaders and social media to engage the public with trustworthy information; engaging children early on through One Health education in schools.
> - Collecting data on monitoring, evaluation, and performance to inform and strengthen response efforts.

on public health capacities and highlighted the need for international monitoring to generate data on this spending. Risk communication also warrants more attention, he added. He emphasized that agriculture is often absent from the conversation and identified this gap as a blind spot in the One Health arena. Despite widespread acknowledgment of the importance of food security, agriculture recedes to the background outside periods of famine and drought, Kester noted. He suggested a midterm goal of mobilizing communities through education and the concept of citizen scientists, as this can expand surveillance and health literacy beyond physicians and veterinarians to encompass a broader segment of society. Remarking that spending is not always reflective of the efficacy of intervention, Kester highlighted a long-term goal of evaluating interventions with respect to their effectiveness in meeting identified needs. Evaluation data can then be used in a dynamic and continually evolving response process.

Surveillance and Detection Mechanisms

Maureen Lichtveld, dean of the University of Pittsburgh's Graduate School of Public Health, moderated the breakout discussion on surveillance and detection mechanisms, which focused on the availability and quality of data and their use in decision making (see Box 7-2). She outlined

---

BOX 7-2
Highlights from Discussion on Surveillance and Detection Mechanisms

Presented by Maureen Lichtveld, University of Pittsburgh

Activities to support primary focus on data acquisition and use:
- Enhancing the availability of local-level data by implementing reliable diagnostic testing to support surveillance systems and building a harmonized platform for rapid reporting and sharing.
- Developing the capacity to use data tools effectively at the higher level to understand the current landscape and determine which decisions can be made reliably based on the data.

Short-term strategic imperatives:
- Funding basic research to build data tools.
- Creating a government structure for One Health surveillance to coordinate efforts, build trust, and work across sectors.
- Building outreach for global networks and widening sources of data: for example, conduct participatory surveillance, build mobile tools, and ensure that they are broadly available.

Long-term strategic imperatives:
- Creating an integrative surveillance system using smart and new technologies (e.g., artificial intelligence, remote sensing, social media monitoring).
- Integrating sequencing; mainstream other molecular or novel epidemiology approaches.

Immediate feasible actions:
- Engaging agencies that work with wildlife and environmental monitoring (e.g., U.S. Geological Survey, other federal and state agencies responsible for natural resources).
- Integrating and expanding species-agnostic approaches to monitoring diseases across humans, livestock, household animals, and urban wildlife.

several goals that participants identified. The first goal is to establish a wide-reaching surveillance system that collects data from disparate silo-driven systems and amasses them into a single global platform. Second, a single, integrated information technology platform could extend beyond single systems and traditional data to create an iterative surveillance system that incorporates data from social media and citizen science input. By creating a system in which data improve in quality while being operationalized locally, local-level public health can become the locus of both decision making and decision implementation. This involves investing time in surveillance systems before an outbreak occurs, rather than waiting until the response phase, said Lichtveld. Third, an opportunity for surveillance innovation exists within low- and middle-income countries, which tend to be less burdened by silo-driven approaches to surveillance and detection than high-income countries. She noted that the breakout group emphasized the importance of communication in integrating participatory surveillance.

Forecasting and Predictive Innovations

Peter Daszak, president at EcoHealth Alliance, moderated the breakout group discussion on forecasting and predictive innovations and outlined three action areas identified (see Box 7-3). First, improvements in data collection and use are needed. A shareable pipeline of real-time genomic data could enable integrating predictive innovations into routine practice. Despite substantial challenges in this area, advances could result in better datasets on human activities. Furthermore, insufficient data on the wildlife trade could be augmented. Low-level collection efforts could result in acceptable data without a public sense of privacy invasion.

Second, education and culture can be used as avenues for strengthening One Health. Education efforts at the primary and secondary levels can help the public understand the value of One Health initiatives and engender support for funding. Moreover, a critical need exists at the postsecondary level for inter-professional education that incorporates data analytics, law, and economics into One Health education, said Daszak. Building centers of interdisciplinary excellence would help address this need. Regarding culture, prioritized values should shift from focusing on per-capita health care spending to valuing health and drivers of health, such as nature, biodiversity, and ecosystem services. Developing a deeper understanding of these factors could increase appreciation for the value of One Health issues, leading to improved global health systems equipped to identify and respond appropriately to first cases and small outbreaks.

Third, predictive approaches should move beyond academia to practical application to achieve impact, said Daszak. Policy makers commonly push back on innovative, predictive approaches, particularly if they lack

> **BOX 7-3**
> **Highlights from Discussion on
> Forecasting and Predictive Innovations**
>
> *Presented by Peter Daszak, EcoHealth Alliance*
>
> Innovations to improve data collection and use:
> - Leveraging the genomic data pipeline and sharing capacity.
> - Developing better datasets on human activities at the interface of One Health.
> - Broadening the collection of low-level data that are societally acceptable.
>
> Innovations in education and culture:
> - Expanding inter-professional education (e.g., data analytics, law in One Health, economics).
> - Building centers of interdisciplinary excellence.
> - Exploring how society values health and drivers of health, including biodiversity, ecosystem services, and nature.
> - Improving health systems to better prevent the escalation of crisis events.
> - Increasing food security and addressing root causes of risks.
>
> Use predictive approaches to move beyond "firefighting":
> - Quantifying risk more accurately and working creatively with disparate data.
> - Making predictions that are useful to policy and agencies (e.g., focus on geography and surveillance targets).
> - Identifying which microbes are most likely to emerge next and developing triage approaches.
> - Conducting genomic analysis of specific sites of interest using real-time data; begin with more predictable microbes (e.g., antimicrobial resistance genes, coronavirus spike proteins).
> - Optimizing use of wearable and sensor technologies.

confidence in the accuracy of prediction capability and feel comfortable with the status quo. To achieve real change, researchers should improve the ability to quantify risk, work creatively with insufficient or inadequate datasets, and make predictions that are useful to policy makers and agencies in terms of geographic focus or targeted species. If researchers are able to identify ever-higher numbers of microbes, a universal system will be needed to triage by importance. Daszak suggested prioritizing microbes for which prediction capability already exists, such as antimicrobial resistance genes and coronaviruses. Finally, given the growth of wearable and sensor technologies linked to smartphones, these are an underused resource that could increase prediction capability, particularly in regions where new diseases are emerging.

DISCUSSION

Social Sciences in One Health

Given that greater incorporation of social sciences would benefit One Health, Mazet asked how social scientists can be included in One Health initiatives. Catherine Machalaba, senior policy advisor and senior scientist at EcoHealth Alliance, noted that One Health is context specific, so the context, community, and scale of an initiative will inform which partners may be relevant. Areas that would benefit from the contribution of social science perspectives include behavioral economics and the design of appropriate community-engagement interventions. For example, the PREDICT project's book, *Living Safely with Bats*,[1] was designed as a visual tool to engage communities about their consumptive practices and exposures and introduce practical solutions. This type of work—involving social scientists, artists, and other professionals outside the major One Health disciplines—could be helpful if introduced on a broader scale.

Olga Jonas, research associate at Harvard University, suggested that efforts should focus on strengthening data collection systems to improve worldwide surveillance, diagnostic, and analytic capacities. She noted that behavior drives the lack of prevention and ultimate costs of outbreaks. Even in wealthy countries, data collection and modeling performed by people who lack sufficient expertise can undermine response efforts and public health as a whole, said Jonas. She remarked that strengthening basic data systems and enabling accurate analysis would encourage constructive public engagement.

Brianna Skinner, senior regulatory veterinarian at the U.S. Food and Drug Administration (FDA), emphasized that social drivers affect all sectors. Human behavior affects the climate, human habitats, the soil used for agriculture, and more. Therefore, FDA is working to diversify One Health personnel beyond biologists, veterinarians, and physicians to create a One Health strategy to help shape public attitudes and behaviors to benefit people, animals, and the environment. FDA is using the One Health concept to address public health issues within its purview; to this end, it has created a One Health steering committee to issue policy, guidance, and standards, said Skinner.

Economic Drivers

Noting the importance of economic impact on health outcomes and the value of economic drivers for healthy behaviors, Mazet asked about

---

[1] More information about *Living Safely with Bats* can be found at https://p2.predict.global/living-safely-with-bats-book (accessed April 28, 2021).

the roles of socioeconomics experts, the World Trade Organization (WTO), and the International Monetary Fund (IMF) in One Health efforts. Laura Kahn, research scholar at the Program on Science and Global Security at the Woodrow Wilson School of Public and International Affairs, Princeton University, remarked that behavioral and sociological activities drive pandemics. To address root causes of these behaviors, society needs to reassess the value of nature and natural resources. Presently, a nation's wealth is typically measured by its gross domestic product (GDP), but this narrow metric only considers a nation's annual output of products and services. She posited that it should also include factors such as water purity, air clarity, soil condition, health of flora and fauna, and ecosystem diversity—all of which affect food security and population health. Exemplifying this more holistic perspective, a group in China developed the concept of the "gross ecosystem product" to serve as a substitute for GDP (Ouyang et al., 2020). By using such a metric, One Health could contribute data and analysis to supplement the GDP and present a more accurate picture of a nation's health landscape, said Kahn. Engaging economists and WTO and IMF in this work could increase the value placed on natural resources; this, in turn, might help prevent events that devastate the global economy.

Mainstreaming the One Health Concept

Mazet stated that for approximately four decades, One Health has largely remained an academic concept. Operationalization began when professional organizations implemented One Health approaches, with momentum now emerging within the private sector and pharmaceutical industry. However, because health effects affect everyone, Mazet asked how the concept might become more mainstreamed among taxpayers. Barbara Han, disease ecologist at Cary Institute of Ecosystem Studies, remarked that COVID-19 has provided an opportunity for One Health practitioners to share expertise with the public in an accessible way. She suggested that the public is now less likely to question the relevance of this work than before the pandemic began, when much of them did not understand the value of sequencing viruses to establish a baseline to assess risk. These challenging concepts are easier to comprehend within the pandemic context, as are the costs of failing to invest in virus research, she noted. Han emphasized that the health community needs to stay committed to this message now that people are actively listening.

Andrew Maccabe, chief executive officer at the American Association of Veterinary Medical Colleges, noted the ongoing challenge of breaking down barriers to integrate One Health beyond specialists and scientists. He added that even within one's own profession, communication can be difficult; hence, effectively communicating with the public can be daunting. Highlighting the National Academy of Medicine's initiative integrating humanities and the arts with science, education, and medicine, Maccabe stated that the more engagement artists and people in the humanities have with these topics, the more likely connections about global health will enter the collective consciousness (NASEM, 2018).

Michael Wilkes, professor of internal medicine at UC Davis suggested starting downstream by integrating One Health concepts into the educational system, strengthening health literacy and numeracy to foster public understanding of the interrelationships between humans, animals, agriculture, and the environment. Moreover, in addition to a presence across traditional and social media outlets, Wilkes remarked on the need for greater dissemination of information in communities that have been underserved during the COVID-19 pandemic. He posited that disparities in testing, infection, and vaccination in some communities reflect the health community's limited ability to communicate and build trust with all communities. He suggested engaging more robustly with stakeholders in these underserved communities.

Mazet recounted discussion earlier in the workshop regarding the incorporation of One Health lessons into grade-school education, similar to the successful recycling curriculum implemented in the past. She recalled an iconic television commercial from the 1970s, in which an Indigenous person was saddened by littering, which had a profound impact on her in instilling the value of not littering. Mazet remarked that One Health needs to create a similar iconic moment. Jonathan Sleeman, director at the U.S. Geological Survey's National Wildlife Health Center, commented that the COVID-19 pandemic is a transformative moment. The definition of One Health speaks to optimizing outcomes for humans, animals, and the environment; however, defining those optimal outcomes is a question not of science but rather of societal value. He suggested that the One Health community should clearly articulate a core set of values—such as maintaining the integrity of natural ecosystems, preserving biodiversity, and advancing equity and food security—and then educate the public on those values.

Lichtveld stressed that progress in incorporating One Health into the mainstream hinges on the ability to translate data into action at the local level, as well as on investing in local public health infrastructure. The One Health movement should address the root causes of disparities that leave some parents facing decisions such as whether to buy food or an inhaler for their child with asthma. Lichtveld shared a vision wherein One Health engages communities as partners—not as subjects—and creates an environment in which community members act as One Health messengers, rather than government representatives. Furthermore, community participatory strategies can serve to extend the reach of One Health and simultaneously make it better understood. Investing in local public health infrastructure should be integral to One Health efforts, Lichtveld added.

Claire Standley, professor at the Center for Global Health Science and Security at Georgetown University, pointed out that the One Health concept is not new: it has long been routinely practiced by Indigenous societies and people living close to wildlife. These communities can meaningfully contribute to the ongoing dialogue, with One Health practitioners learning from their examples and experience. Kaylee Myhre Errecaborde, policy researcher and veterinarian at the University of Minnesota College of Veterinary Medicine, noted that despite collaborative advantage, collaborative inertia can occur, impeding the process of prioritizing participants to the specific issue at hand. Collaboration requires considerable energy and resources, but prioritizing the participants who are most critical to each conversation or technical activity can help to maximize the impact of collaborative efforts.

Tracey McNamara, professor at the College of Veterinary Medicine at Western University of Health Sciences, highlighted a common misconception that the U.S. Department of Agriculture oversees all national surveillance of zoonotic threats. Efforts to increase public awareness are needed, because the public is largely unaware of the hierarchies involved in One Health surveillance in the United States and the substantial gaps in it. She noted that funding allocation—which often designates all funds to a single agency—can result in conflicts that impede collaboration and progress of One Health surveillance. To limit interagency conflicts, McNamara suggested a concept where each participating agency votes on how funding is allocated. She also emphasized the value of public engagement in advocating for legislative changes. Mazet added that the siloing in the structure of the U.S. government is an additional barrier to collaboration.

Daszak commented on the public's lack of knowledge about global health concerns. He noted the critical role that popular interest efforts can play in raising awareness of the threat of outbreaks, such as the *Outbreak: Epidemics in a Connected World* exhibit,[2] the film *Contagion* (Soderbergh, 2011), and a recent episode of *Last Week Tonight* with John Oliver, "The Next Pandemic" (Pennolino and Werner, 2021). A lack of education about outbreak sources at the middle- and high-school levels has contributed to disbelief that COVID-19 was caused by nature, which, in turn, fuels vaccine hesitancy, said Daszak. He suggested that viruses and public health issues be added to secondary school curricula to leverage the current receptive state of the general public. Furthermore, he stressed that in order to solicit public involvement, scientists should be explicit in highlighting the human role in environmental problems—and, in turn, health concerns—and in creating solutions to these human-made issues. Messaging that appeals to

---

[2] More information about this exhibit can be found at https://naturalhistory.si.edu/exhibits/outbreak-epidemics-connected-world (accessed April 28, 2021).

emotion in connecting humans to the natural environment can be effective in changing behavior, as was the case with the conservation campaigns of the 1960s and 1970s.

Peter Rabinowitz, professor and director of the Center for One Health Research at the University of Washington, echoed the idea that the COVID-19 pandemic is an opportunity for restructuring systems in accordance with One Health principles. In addition, opportunities exist to harness young people's current enthusiasm for addressing climate change and eradicating institutionalized racism toward expanding the One Health approach. One Health practitioners can capitalize on these opportunities by raising awareness of the connections between One Health, climate change, and the impacts of racism on social determinants of health, said Rabinowitz. John Amuasi emphasized that the One Health movement should extend beyond research and academia to incorporate activism. He added that climate change scientists have been more successful in soliciting public support than have researchers in other areas, which is likely attributable to their engagement with activism. Furthermore, he noted the Black Lives Matter movement has had a greater impact on shifting institutional racism in a relatively short period of time than have research and academic efforts. Given the close ties of racial health disparities and climate change with the One Health approach, activism can serve as an effective vehicle for expanding the One Health platform, said Amuasi.

Ben Beard, deputy division director of the U.S. Centers for Disease Control and Prevention (CDC) Division of Vector-Borne Diseases, suggested that efforts should focus on coordinating systems that are already in place, rather than creating a One Health surveillance system. He pointed out that state governments—not the federal government—are responsible for national surveillance, with the Council of State and Territorial Epidemiologists serving as the governing body and CDC coordinating these efforts. Data-use agreements and concerns around personally identifiable information pose challenges to public health coordination with other agencies, yet this collaboration is necessary and must be strengthened, said Beard. Furthermore, climate change is a pressing concern that requires efforts to expand from disease surveillance to include forecasting. Models can integrate surveillance data and are capable of providing faster responses than traditional surveillance data methods. For example, the public health response to local outbreaks of West Nile virus typically begins as the outbreak is ending. Beard linked this to insufficient forecasting tools and inadequate capacity to convince the public to take prevention steps before an outbreak spreads.

Kahn spoke about the need to include microbial education in gradeschool curriculum. As the world is microbial and the human body is largely composed of microbes, people can learn to move more safely in their communities by learning how to prevent the spread of dangerous microbes between one another, animals, and the environment. Such education efforts could prove helpful in preventing disease outbreaks, said Kahn.

Marc Allard, research microbiologist and senior advisor for genomics at FDA's Center for Food Safety and Applied Nutrition, stressed the importance of collaborating with state and academic partners, the Department of Health and Human Services, and USDA. Sharing tools and broad communication of standard operating procedures for any stage—be it collecting the isolates, sequencing the isolates, uploading the data, or interpreting the data—empowers partners and fosters communication at the national and international levels. Furthermore, shared protocols and tools enable the establishment of standard, validated methods, enabling efficiency and efficacy, said Smolinski.

Collaborations in Moving Forward

Casey Barton Behravesh, director of the One Health office at CDC, underscored the value of collaboration and identified One Health coordination as a key component in successes achieved during the COVID-19 pandemic. She cited the 2017 collaboration between CDC, the U.S. Department of the Interior, USDA, and multiple other agencies and departments. The collective group developed a list of prioritized zoonotic disease threats in the United States, in which coronaviruses ranked fifth.[3] Noting action plans to promote One Health, she highlighted 2021 legislation that directs the federal government to create a national One Health framework to combat the threat of zoonotic diseases, advance emergency preparedness, and establish a formalized One Health coordination mechanism at the federal level.[4] Barton Behravesh stated that if passed into law, this legislation will be critically important in fostering interagency collaboration, focusing on shared priorities, and creating a unified framework to demonstrate the needed steps and resources—including a dedicated budget line for One Health activities—to tackle these issues and better serve the collective health goals of the nation.

Mazet remarked that many One Health practitioners have slowly and steadily made inroads in advancing this approach over several decades, but the COVID-19 pandemic has catalyzed momentum toward changing not only the way health problem solving is approached but the very way humans function on Earth. She noted that it is only one of the multiple syndemics—the synergistic interactions between socioecological and

---

[3] More information about this workshop is available at https://www.cdc.gov/onehealth/what-we-do/zoonotic-disease-prioritization/us-workshops.html (accessed May 28, 2021).

[4] Advancing Emergency Preparedness Through One Health Act of 2021, S.861, 117th Cong., 1st sess. (March 18, 2021).

biological factors that result in adverse health outcomes—the world is facing. Addressing these syndemics will require pulling together diverse thoughts, experiences, and social contexts to generate new ideas, research, and solutions that are palatable to the global community, said Mazet. She emphasized that One Health has the potential to serve in this capacity, but only if equity, inclusion, and diversity are valued and the voices of people facing the greatest adverse health outcomes are spotlighted. Accomplishing this paradigm shift will require leadership and advocacy in all directions and opening national and disciplinary boundaries, she noted. Finally, Mazet acknowledged that as all things are connected, humans must connect their ideas; no individual or discipline is capable of solving these problems alone.

References

Aberdeenshire Community Planning Partnership, and What Works Scotland. 2018. Inquiring into multi-layered, preventative partnership working. http://whatworksscotland.ac.uk/wp-content/uploads/2018/03/InquiringIntoMulti-layeredPreventativePartnershipWorking.pdf (accessed April 21, 2021).

Allen, A. T. 2010. You have to lead from everywhere. Interviewed by Scott Berinato. *Harvard Business Review* 88(11):76-79, 149.

Allen, T., K. A. Murray, C. Zambrana-Torrelio, S. S. Morse, C. Rondinini, M. Di Marco, N. Breit, K. J. Olival, and P. Daszak. 2017. Global hotspots and correlates of emerging zoonotic diseases. *Nature Communications* 8(1):1-10.

Amuasi, J. H., T. Lucas, R. Horton, and A. S. Winkler. 2020a. Reconnecting for our future: The Lancet One Health Commission. *Lancet* 395(10235):1469-1471.

Amuasi, J. H., C. Walzer, D. Heymann, H. Carabin, L. T. Huong, A. Haines, and A. S. Winkler. 2020b. Calling for a COVID-19 One Health research coalition. *Lancet* 395(10236):1543-1544.

Beeston, C., G. McCarney, J. Ford, E. Wimbush, S. Beck, W. MacDonald, and A. Fraser. 2014. *Health inequalities policy review for the Scottish Ministerial Task Force on Health Inequalities.* Edinburgh, Scotland: NHS Health Scotland.

Bhattacharya, S. 2008. The World Health Organization and global smallpox eradication. *Journal of Epidemiology & Community Health* 62:909-912.

Binagwaho, A., and K. Mathewos. 2020. *Opinion: Why universal health coverage is the key to pandemic management.* https://www.devex.com/news/opinion-why-universal-health-coverage-is-the-key-to-pandemic-management-98345 (accessed September 30, 2021).

Bogich, T. L., R. Chunara, D. Scales, E. Chan, L. C. Pinheiro, A. A. Chmura, D. Carroll, P. Daszak, and J. S. Brownstein. 2012. Preventing pandemics via international development: A systems approach. *PLOS Medicine* 9(12):e1001354.

CDC (U.S. Centers for Disease Control and Prevention). 2018. *One Health Basics.* Centers for Disease Control and Prevention. https://www.cdc.gov/onehealth/basics/index.html (accessed September 30, 2021).

Daszak, P., C. das Neves, J. Amuasi, D. Hayman, T. Kuiken, B. Roche, C. Zambrana-Torrelio, P. Buss, H. Dundarova, Y. Feferholtz, G. Foldvari, E. Igbinosa, S. Junglen, Q. Liu, G. Suzan, M. Uhart, C. Wannous, K. Woolaston, P. Mosig Reidl, K. O'Brien, U. Pascual, P. Stoett, H. Li, and H. T. Ngo. 2020. *IPBES (2020) workshop report on biodiversity and pandemics of the intergovernmental platform on biodiversity and ecosystem services.* Bonn, Germany: IPBES Secretariat.

Dos S. Ribeiro, C., L. van de Burgwal, and B. J. Regeer. 2019. Overcoming challenges for designing and implementing the One Health approach: A systematic review of the literature. *One Health* 7:100085. https://doi.org/10.1016/j.onehlt.2019.100085.

Emanuel, R. 2020. Let's make sure this crisis doesn't go to waste. *The Washington Post*, March 25. https://www.washingtonpost.com/opinions/2020/03/25/lets-make-sure-this-crisis-doesnt-go-waste (accessed September 30, 2021).

Ge, X. Y., N. Wang, W. Zhang, B. Hu, B. Li, Y. Z. Zhang, J. H. Zhou, C. M. Luo, X. L. Yang, L. J. Wu, B. Wang, Y. Zhang, Z. X. Li, and Z. L. Shi. 2016. Coexistence of multiple coronaviruses in several bat colonies in an abandoned mineshaft. *Virological Sinica* 31(1):31-40.

Graham, B. S., and N. J. Sullivan. 2018. Emerging viral diseases from a vaccinology perspective: Preparing for the next pandemic. *Nature Immunology* 19(1):20-28.

Hale, T., N. Angrist, R. Goldszmidt, B. Kira, A. Petherick, T. Phillips, S. Webster, E. Cameron-Blake, L. Hallas, and S. Majumdar. 2021. A global panel database of pandemic policies (Oxford COVID-19 government response tracker). *Nature Human Behaviour* 5(4):529-538.

Holligan, A. 2021. *COVID: Dutch curfew riots rage for third night.* BBC News. https://www.bbc.com/news/world-europe-55799919 (accessed January 20, 2022).

IOM (Institute of Medicine). 2004. *Learning from SARS: Preparing for the next disease outbreak: Workshop summary.* Washington, DC: The National Academies Press.

Kanter, R. M. 2020. *Think outside the building: How advanced leaders can change the world one smart innovation at a time.* New York: PublicAffairs.

Karim, N., L. Jing, J. A. Lee, R. Kharel, D. Lubetkin, C. M. Clancy, D. Uwamahoro, E. Nahayo, J. Biramahire, A. R. Aluisio, and V. Ndebwanimana. 2021. Lessons Learned from Rwanda: Innovative strategies for prevention and containment of COVID-19. *Annals of Global Health* 87(1):23.

Link, B. G., and J. Phelan. 1995. Social conditions as fundamental causes of disease. *Journal of Health and Social Behavior* Spec No:80-94.

Marcus, L. J., B. C. Dorn, and J. M. Henderson. 2006. Meta-leadership and national emergency preparedness: A model to build government connectivity. *Biosecurity and Bioterrorism* 4(2):128-134.

Marcus, J. L., W. A. Leyden, S. E. Alexeeff, A. N. Anderson, R. C. Hechter, H. Hu, J. O. Lam, W. J. Towner, Q. Yuan, M. A. Horberg, and M. J. Silverberg. 2020. Comparison of overall and comorbidity-free life expectancy between insured adults with and without HIV infection, 2000–2016. *JAMA Network Open* 3(6):e207954.

Mason-D'Croz, D., J. R. Bogard, M. Herrero, S. Robinson, T. B. Sulser, K. Wiebe, D. Willenbockel, and H. C. J. Godfray. 2020. Modelling the global economic consequences of a major African swine fever outbreak in China. *Nature Food* 1(4):221-228.

Mawathe, A. 2021. *COVAX vaccine-sharing scheme delivers first doses to Ghana.* BBC News. https://www.bbc.com/news/world-africa-56180161 (accessed January 20, 2022).

Mutesa, L., P. Ndshimye, Y. Butera, J. Souopgui, A. Uwineza, R. Rutayisire, E. L. Ndoricimpaye, E. Musoni, N. Rujeni, T. Nyatanyi, E. Ntagwabira, M. Semakula, C. Musanabaganwa, D. Nyamwasa, M. Ndashimye, E. Ujeneza, I. E. Mwikarago, C. M. Muvunyi, J. B. Mazarati, S. Nsanzimana, N. Turok, and W. Ndifon. 2021. A pooled testing strategy for identifying SARS-CoV-2 at low prevalence. *Nature* 589(7841):276-280.

NASEM (National Academies of Sciences, Engineering, and Medicine). 2018. *The integration of the humanities and arts with sciences, engineering, and medicine in higher education: Branches from the same tree.* Washington, DC: The National Academies Press.

NASEM. 2019a. *The convergence of infectious diseases and noncommunicable diseases: Proceedings of a workshop.* Washington, DC: The National Academies Press.

NASEM. 2019b. *Exploring lessons learned from a century of outbreaks: Readiness for 2030: Proceedings of a workshop.* Washington, DC: The National Academies Press

NASEM. 2020. *Exploring the frontiers of innovation to tackle microbial threats: Proceedings of a workshop.* Washington, DC: The National Academies Press.

Nyamusore, J., J. B. Mazarati, P. Ndimubanzi, A. Kabeja, H. Balisanga, F. Nizeyimana, L. Ruyange, A. Kapiteni, I. Itanga, V. Ndagijimana, M. Gashegu, S. Uwamahoro, C. Murekatete, A. Umutoni, C. Nsanzabaganwa, N. Hitimana, F. Byiringiro, S. Nsanzimana, L. Mutesa, and D. Gashumba. 2019. The Rwanda national Ebola preparedness exercise and response strategies. *Rwanda Public Health Bulletin* 1(2):6-10.

Nyatanyi, T., M. Wilkes, H. McDermott, S. Nzietchueng, I. Gafarasi, A. Mudakikwa, J. F. Kinani, J. Rukelibuga, J. Omolo, D. Mupfasoni, A. Kabeja, J. Nyamusore, J. Nziza, J. L. Hakizimana, J. Kamugisha, R. Nkunda, R. Kibuuka, E. Rugigana, P. Farmer, P. Cotton, and A. Binagwaho. 2017. Implementing One Health as an integrated approach to health in Rwanda. *BMJ Global Health* 2(1):e000121.

OIE (World Organisation for Animal Health). 2012. *OIE recommendations on the competencies of graduating veterinarians ("day 1 graduates") to assure national veterinary services of quality.* World Organisation for Animal Health. https://www.oie.int/fileadmin/Home/eng/Support_to_OIE_Members/Vet_Edu_AHG/DAY_1/DAYONE-B-ang-vC.pdf (accessed September 30, 2021).

OIE. 2019a. *Aquatic animal health code, 22nd edition.* World Organisation for Animal Health. https://rr-europe.oie.int/wp-content/uploads/2020/08/oie-aqua-code_2019_en.pdf (accessed September 30, 2021).

OIE. 2019b. *Terrestrial animal health code, 28th edition.* World Organisation for Animal Health. https://rr-europe.oie.int/wp-content/uploads/2020/08/oie-terrestrial-code-1_2019_en.pdf (accessed September 30, 2021).

OIE. 2020. *Global Situation of African Swine Fever.* World Organisation for Animal Health. https://www.oie.int/app/uploads/2021/03/report-47-global-situation-asf.pdf (accessed September 30, 2021).

O'Neill, J. 2016. *Tackling drug-resistant infections globally: Final report and recommendations.* Review on Antimicrobial Resistance. https://amr-review.org/sites/default/files/160518_Final%20paper_with%20cover.pdf (accessed November 30, 2021).

Ouyang, Z., C. Song, H. Zheng, S. Polasky, Y. Xiao, I. J. Bateman, J. Liu, M. Ruckelshaus, F. Shi, Y. Xiao, W. Xu, Z. Zou, and G. C. Daily. 2020. Using gross ecosystem product (GEP) to value nature in decision making. *Proceedings of the National Academy of Sciences* 117(25):14593-14601.

Pennolino, P., and C. Werner. 2021. *Last Week Tonight with John Oliver. The Next Pandemic.* https://www.hbo.com/last-week-tonight-with-john-oliver/season-8/1-february-14-2021-next-pandemic (accessed January 14, 2022).

PREDICT Consortium. 2020. *Advancing Global Health Security at the Frontiers of Disease Emergence.* One Health Institute, University of California, Davis.

Reid, M., Q. Abdool-Karim, E. Geng, and E. Goosby. 2021. *How will COVID-19 transform global health post-pandemic? Defining research and investment opportunities and priorities.* San Francisco, CA: Public Library of Science.

Review on Antimicrobial Resistance. 2015. *Securing new drugs for future generations: The pipeline of antibiotics.* Review on Antimicrobial Resistance. https://amr-review.org/sites/default/files/SECURING%20NEW%20DRUGS%20FOR%20FUTURE%20GENERATIONS%20FINAL%20WEB_0.pdf (accessed September 30, 2021).

Rose, G. 1985. Sick individuals and sick populations. *International Journal of Epidemiology* 14(1):32-38.

Rosenberg, R., N. P. Lindsey, M. Fischer, C. J. Gregory, A. F. Hinckley, P. S. Mead, G. Paz-Bailey, S. H. Waterman, N. A. Drexler, G. J. Kersh, H. Hooks, S. K. Partridge, S. N. Visser, C. B. Beard, and L. R. Petersen. 2018. Vital signs: Trends in reported vectorborne disease cases—United States and territories, 2004–2016. *Morbidity and Mortality Weekly Report* 67(17):496-501.

Sharp, P., S. Hockfield, and T. Jacks. 2016. *Convergence: The future of health.* Cambridge, MA: Massachusetts Institute of Technology.

Soderbergh, S. 2011. *Contagion.* United States: Warner Bros. Pictures.

Solomon, S. L., and K. B. Oliver. 2014. Antibiotic resistance threats in the United States: Stepping back from the brink. *American Family Physician* 89(12):938-941.

Spellberg, B., J. G. Bartlett, and D. N. Gilbert. 2013. The future of antibiotics and resistance. *New England Journal of Medicine* 368(4):299-302.

Swanson, A. 2018. Trump's trade war with China is officially underway. *The New York Times,* July 6, B1.

Taylor, L. H., S. M. Latham, and M. E. Woolhouse. 2001. Risk factors for human disease emergence. *Philosophical Transactions of the Royal Society of London. Series B, Biological Sciences* 356(1411):983-989.

Thompson, C. 2018. Rose's prevention paradox. *Journal of Applied Philosophy* 35(2):242-256.

Togami, E., J. L. Gardy, G. R. Hansen, G. H. Poste, D. M. Rizzo, M. E. Wilson, and J. A. K. Mazet. 2018. Core competencies in One Health education: What are we missing? *NAM Perspectives.* Discussion Paper, National Academy of Medicine, Washington, DC. https://doi.org/10.31478/201806a (accessed January 20, 2022).

Wacharapluesadee, S., C. W. Tan, P. Maneeorn, P. Duengkae, F. Zhu, Y. Joyjinda, T. Kaewpom, W. N. Chia, W. Ampoot, B. L. Lim, K. Worachotsueptrakun, V. C. Chen, N. Sirichan, C. Ruchisrisarod, A. Rodpan, K. Noradechanon, T. Phaichana, N. Jantarat, B. Thongnumchaima, C. Tu, G. Crameri, M. M. Stokes, T. Hemachudha, and L. F. Wang. 2021. Evidence for SARS-COV-2 related coronaviruses circulating in bats and pangolins in Southeast Asia. *Nature Communications* 12(1):972.

Wane, J., T. Nyatanyi, R. Nkunda, J. Rukelibuga, Z. Ahmed, C. Biedron, A. Kabeja, M. A. Muhimpundu, A. Kabanda, S. Antara, O. Briet, J. B. Koama, A. Rusanganwa, O. Mukabayire, C. Karema, P. Raghunathan, and D. Lowrance. 2012. 2009 pandemic influenza a (H1NI) virus outbreak and response—Rwanda, October, 2009–May, 2010. *PLoS One* 7(6):e31572.

WHO (World Health Organization). 2008a. *International health regulations (2005).* Geneva, Switzerland: World Health Organization.

WHO. 2008b. *International health regulations (2005) second edition.* Geneva, Switzerland: World Health Organization.

WHO. 2014. *Antimicrobial resistance: Global report on surveillance.* Geneva, Switzerland: World Health Organization.

WHO. 2018. *Managing epidemics: Key facts about major deadly diseases.* Geneva, Switzerland: World Health Organization.

WHO. 2020. *Guidance for conducting a country COVID-19 intra-action review, 23 July 2020.* Geneva, Switzerland: World Health Organization.

Wilson, J. 2020. US lockdown protests may have spread virus widely, cellphone data suggests. *The Guardian*, May 18, https://www.theguardian.com/us-news/2020/may/18/lockdown-protests-spread-coronavirus-cellphone-data (accessed September 30, 2021).

World Bank Group. 2018. *One health: Operational framework for strengthening human, animal, and environmental public health systems at their interface.* Washington, DC: The World Bank.

Zaki, A. M., S. van Boheemen, T. M. Bestebroer, A. D. Osterhaus, and R. A. Fouchier. 2012. Isolation of a novel coronavirus from a man with pneumonia in Saudi Arabia. *New England Journal of Medicine* 367(19):1814-1820.

Zhou, P., X. L. Yang, X. G. Wang, B. Hu, L. Zhang, W. Zhang, H. R. Si, Y. Zhu, B. Li, C. L. Huang, H. D. Chen, J. Chen, Y. Luo, H. Guo, R. D. Jiang, M. Q. Liu, Y. Chen, X. R. Shen, X. Wang, X. S. Zheng, K. Zhao, Q. J. Chen, F. Deng, L. L. Liu, B. Yan, F. X. Zhan, Y. Y. Wang, G. F. Xiao, and Z. L. Shi. 2020. A pneumonia outbreak associated with a new coronavirus of probable bat origin. *Nature* 579(7798):270-273.

Appendix A

Workshop Statement of Task

A planning committee of the National Academies of Sciences, Engineering, and Medicine will organize a workshop to examine ways to systemize and integrate the One Health approach as part of outbreak prevention, detection, preparedness, and response efforts. The in-person workshop will explore research opportunities, multi-sectoral collaboration mechanisms, community engagement strategies, educational opportunities, and policies that can effectively implement the core capacities and interventions of One Health principles to strengthen national health systems and enhance global health security.

Specifically, the workshop will feature invited presentations and discussions on the following topics:

- Strategies to build a strong investment case to overcome political and technical impasses to systematize One Health in national prevention, detection, preparedness, and response efforts;
- Evaluation of One Health programs integrated into national and global public health efforts;
- Integration of animal and human health surveillance systems for cross-reporting to better understand pathogens in animals before (or after) spill-over to humans;
- Feasibility of introducing and integrating One Health into existing coordination mechanisms, and into national action plans based on the Joint External Evaluation;
- Strengthening the global health workforce with One Health capacities;

- Policies that underscore the interconnectedness of animal, human, and environmental health;
- Implications of using a One Health approach to improve preparedness versus a reactionary response that is required to create medical countermeasures after outbreak onset;
- Best practices for engaging with communities and influencing behaviors that lower the risk of infectious disease infection through the One Health approach;
- The tension between public health needs, the private sector, and data sharing within the One Health context in preparedness and response efforts; and
- Potential priority actions to unite organizations—public and private, domestic and international—in efforts to overcome newly discovered hurdles based on lessons learned from the COVID-19 pandemic.

Speakers and discussants will contribute perspectives from government, academia, private, and nonprofit sectors. The planning committee will organize the workshop, select and invite speakers and discussants, and moderate the discussions. A proceedings of the presentations and discussions will be prepared by a designated rapporteur in accordance with institutional guidelines.

Appendix B

Workshop Agenda

DAY 1 – TUESDAY, 23 February 2021
10:00 am – 1:00 pm

10:00 AM   Welcome Remarks, Workshop Overview, and Goals

Workshop Co-Chairs

CASEY BARTON BEHRAVESH
Director, One Health Office
U.S. Centers for Disease Control and Prevention

JONNA MAZET
Professor of Epidemiology and Disease Ecology
Founding Executive Director, One Health Institute
School of Veterinary Medicine
University of California, Davis

10:10 AM   <u>Keynote Address</u>

"Rx One Health: A Prescription to Prevent Pandemics"
ERIC GOOSBY
Professor of Medicine, University of California, San Francisco, School of Medicine and former United Nations Special Envoy on Tuberculosis

10:40 AM   Q&A

Session I: Defining the One Health State of Affairs

Session I Objectives:
- Assess current One Health programs and efforts worldwide and their participation in the response to global public health crises.
- Showcase how One Health practices have been integrated into existing programs to improve the current model for global public health responses.

> KENT KESTER
> *Session Chair*
> Vice President
> Head, Translational Science and Biomarkers
> Sanofi Pasteur

11:00 AM   **One Health in praxis**

<u>Case Presentations</u>

"Operationalizing One Health at a Local Level"
DANA BECKHAM
Director, Office of Science, Surveillance and Technology
Harris County Public Health, Texas

"Multi-Sectoral Engagement in the COVID-19 Outbreak Response in Thailand"
SUPAPORN WACHARAPLUESADEE
Deputy Chief
Thai Red Cross Emerging Infectious Diseases Health Science Centre

"COVID-19 Response: Lessons Learnt to Reinforce the Relevance of One Health Principles"
THIERRY NYATANYI
Senior Advisor, COVID-19 Taskforce
Africa CDC

12:00 PM   **Q&A**

12:45 PM   **Observations from Day 1**
                  KENT KESTER

1:00 PM   **Adjourn**

APPENDIX B

DAY 2 – WEDNESDAY, 24 February 2021
10:00 am – 1:00 pm

Session II: What Can One Health Do Right Now?

Session II Objectives:
- Assess the current status of developing a One Health workforce to identify gaps between education and training programs and employment needs.
- Explore frameworks to establish cross-sector collaborations and community engagement to strengthen threat surveillance and detection.
- Discuss challenges of and methods for introducing One Health ideology into existing systems for epidemiological surveillance (local, national, international levels).

10:00 AM   Welcome and Recap Day 1
            EVA HARRIS
            Session Chair
            Professor, Division of Infectious Diseases and Vaccinology
            Director, Center for Global Public Health,
            University of California, Berkeley

10:05 AM   Panel Discussions

            Panel I: What Is Being Done Right Now?
            Moderator: Mark Smolinski (Ending Pandemics)

            DAVID GOLDMAN
            JAMES HOSPEDALES
            CARRIE S. McNEIL
            DAVID RIZZO
            ESRON KARIMURIBO

10:35 AM   Q&A

11:00 AM   Panel II: What Could We Be Doing Better?
            Moderator: John Nkengasong (Africa Centres for Disease Control and Prevention)

            JOHN BALBUS
            CHRISTOPHER BRADEN
            CARLOS DAS NEVES
            CRISTINA ROMANELLI

11:30 AM	Q&A
11:55 PM	Break
12:05 PM	Plenary Presentations

<u>I. The One Health Workforce</u>

"One Health Workforce: Reconciling Competencies with Opportunities"
LONNIE KING
Dean Emeritus, College of Veterinary Medicine
The Ohio State University

<u>II. Community Engagement and Frameworks for Collaboration</u>

"University Networks on the Front Lines for Community Engagement and One Health Innovation"
WOUTRINA A. SMITH
Professor, School of Veterinary Medicine
University of California, Davis

12:40 PM	Q&A
12:55 PM	Observations from Day 2 EVA HARRIS
1:00 PM	Adjourn

DAY 3 – THURSDAY, 25 February 2021
10:00 am – 1:00 pm

Session III: Looking Forward – Lessons from the Past and the Future of One Health

Session III Objectives:
- Lessons that can be learned and extrapolated from COVID-19: Priority actions for policy, public-private partnerships, and industry resilience to build a broad, threat-agnostic global health system.
- What comes next: Strategies to facilitate international cooperation and data sharing to establish forecasting capabilities for emerging health threats.

10:00 AM	**Welcome and Recap Day 2** PETER DASZAK *Session Chair* President EcoHealth Alliance
10:05 AM	**Plenary Presentations** *Learning from the past and planning for the future – Collaboration opportunities and priority actions*

<u>I. What future capabilities can we build toward predicting the next outbreak?</u>

"Precision Epidemiology, Human Behavior, and the Future of One Health"

JONATHAN QUICK
Managing Director; Pandemic Response, Preparedness, and Prevention
Health Initiative, The Rockefeller Foundation

<u>II. An example of existing frameworks that could be scaled up to improve public health systems in the United States</u>

"A Collaborative Effort in Outbreak Preparedness: FDA's Approach to African Swine Fever"

DANIELLE SHOLLY and KATHERINE HUEBNER
Animal Scientist, Center for Veterinary Medicine
U.S. Food and Drug Administration

<u>III. What future policies can we develop to support forecasting emerging health threats?</u>

"The Paradox of Global Policies for Pandemic Prediction and Prevention"

JOHN AMUASI
Executive Director
African Research Network for Neglected Tropical Diseases

IV. How can the public and private sectors collaborate to improve resilience against future global health threats?

"Taking Pandemic Threats Off the Table"

RAJEEV VENKAYYA
President, Global Vaccine Business Unit
Takeda Pharmaceuticals

11:05 AM	Q&A
11:30 AM	Break
11:40 PM	Breakout Room Discussions

Key takeaways for building a better system for outbreak response, surveillance/detection, and forecasting
- In-depth discussions that will identify key, feasible goals and steps that can be taken toward improving outbreak preparedness efforts for the future
    - Identify 1-2 short-term goals
    - Identify 1-2 long-term goals
    - Identify key actions and relevant institutions involved in achieving these goals

Breakout 1: Response Capacities
- Moderator: Kent Kester, *Sanofi Pasteur*

- Kaylee Myhre Errecaborde, *University of Minnesota*
- Olga Jonas, *Harvard University*
- Catherine Machalaba, *EcoHealth Alliance*
- Peter Rabinowitz, *University of Washington*
- Michael Wilkes, *University of California, Davis*
- Victor del Rio Vilas, *World Health Organization*

Breakout 2: Surveillance and Detection Mechanisms
- Moderator: Maureen Lichtveld, *University of Pittsburgh*

- Charles (Ben) Beard, *U.S. Centers for Disease Control and Prevention*
- Julie Fischer, *Georgetown University*
- Tracey McNamara, *Western University of Health Sciences*
- Jonathan Sleeman, *U.S. Geological Survey*
- Irene Xagoraraki, *Michigan State University*

Breakout 3: Forecasting and Predictive Innovations
- Moderator: Peter Daszak, *EcoHealth Alliance*

- Marc Allard, *U.S. Food and Drug Administration*
- Greg Glass, *University of Florida*
- Barbara Han, *Cary Institute of Ecosystem Studies*
- Laura Kahn, *Princeton University*
- Andrew Maccabe, *American Association of Veterinary Medical Colleges*
- Claire Standley, *Georgetown University*

12:10 PM	**Breakout Room: Recap**
12:25 PM	**Q&A**
12:55 PM	**Closing Remarks**

Workshop Co-Chairs

CASEY BARTON BEHRAVESH
Director, One Health Office
U.S. Centers for Disease Control and Prevention

JONNA MAZET
Professor of Epidemiology and Disease Ecology
Executive Director, One Health Institute
School of Veterinary Medicine
University of California, Davis

1:00 PM	**Adjourn**

Appendix C

Speaker and Moderator Biographies

Marc Allard, Ph.D., received his doctorate in biology in 1990 from Harvard University. Dr. Allard was the Louis Weintraub Associate Professor of Biology (and Genetics) at George Washington University (Washington, DC) for 14 years from 1994 to 2008. He has had appointments to the Visiting Scientists Program both at the Federal Bureau of Investigation's Counterterrorism and Forensic Science Research Unit and in the Chem.-Bio. Sciences Unit for approximately 8 years, where he assisted in the anthrax investigations as well as in human genetics data-basing. Dr. Allard joined the U.S. Food and Drug Administration (FDA), Office of Regulatory Science, Division of Microbiology in November 2008. He assisted in building FDA's GenomeTrakr Whole Genome Sequencing network for source tracking of foodborne pathogens to rapidly identify outbreaks and the root cause of contamination events for *Salmonella*, *E. coli*, and *Listeria*.

John H. Amuasi, Ph.D., M.P.H., lectures at the Kwame Nkrumah University of Science and Technology (KNUST), where he is based at the Global Health Department of the School of Public Health and is head of the Department of Community Health at the School of Medicine and Dentistry. Dr. Amuasi is also Group Leader of the Global Health and Infectious Diseases Research Group at the Kumasi Center for Collaborative Research in Tropical Medicine (KCCR), which hosts the secretariat of the African Research Network for Neglected Tropical Diseases (ARNTD), of which he is the executive director. Dr. Amuasi trained as a physician at the KNUST School of Medical Sciences, and later graduated from the University of Minnesota School of Public Health, with post-graduate degrees terminating in a Ph.D. in health research and policy. He also served as head of the R&D Unit at the 1,200-bed Komfo Anokye Teaching Hospital in Kumasi, Ghana, from 2007 to 2010. Dr. Amuasi has consulted for several international organizations and is passionate about research that focuses on improving health systems, services, and outcomes, including policy analyses using both primary and secondary data in low- and middle-income countries. His research currently involves field epidemiologic studies on malaria, snakebites, and other neglected tropical diseases. Dr. Amuasi serves as an executive committee member of the African Coalition for Epidemic Research, Response and Training (ALERRT). Through ALERRT at KCCR, Dr. Amuasi is coordinating the setup of research on the clinical characterization of COVID-19 in Africa and is the principal investigator for a number of studies on COVID-19 in Ghana, including a phase III clinical trial. Dr. Amuasi also co-chairs the Lancet One Health Commission and is at the forefront of global efforts toward addressing emerging and re-emerging infectious diseases using a One Health approach.

John Balbus, M.D., M.P.H., serves as a senior advisor and directs the National Institute of Environmental Health Sciences–World Health Organization (NIEHS–WHO) Collaborating Centre for Environmental Health Sciences. He also leads NIEHS efforts on climate change and human health. In this capacity he serves as the U.S. Department of Health and Human Services principal to the U.S. Global Change Research Program, for which he also co-chairs the Interagency Cross-Cutting Group on Climate Change and Human Health. Dr. Balbus's background combines training and experience in clinical medicine with expertise in epidemiology, toxicology, and risk sciences.

Before joining the NIEHS, Dr. Balbus was the chief health scientist for the nongovernmental organization Environmental Defense Fund. He served on the faculty of The George Washington University, where he was founding director of the Center for Risk Science and Public Health, founding co-director of the Mid-Atlantic Center for Children's Health and the Environment, and acting chairman of the Department of Environmental and Occupational Health. He maintains an adjunct faculty appointment at the Milken Institute School of Public Health at The George Washington University. Dr. Balbus received his A.B. degree in biochemistry from Harvard University, his M.D. from the University of Pennsylvania, and his M.P.H. from the Johns Hopkins School of Public Health.

Casey Barton Behravesh, M.S., D.V.M., Dr.P.H., DACVPM (*Co-Chair*), is the director of the U.S. Centers for Disease Control and Prevention's (CDC's) One Health Office in the National Center for Emerging and Zoonotic Infectious Diseases and a captain in the U.S. Public Health Service. Her role is to serve as the agency's lead for implementing a One Health approach to public health that connects human, animal, and environmental health, enabling CDC and partners to address emerging zoonotic and infectious diseases and other shared health threats at the human–animal–environment interface. Dr. Barton Behravesh is experienced in bringing together human, animal, and environmental health officials at the local, state, federal, and global levels to bridge gaps related to emerging zoonotic and infectious diseases, including COVID-19. During her extensive career at CDC, Dr. Barton Behravesh has done everything from investigating outbreaks in the field to conducting epidemiologic research related to the prevention and control of zoonotic, foodborne, and vector-borne diseases. In her leadership role at CDC, she enjoys mentoring students and new staff to help them reach their career goals.

Charles (Ben) Beard, M.S., Ph.D., earned a B.S. in 1980 at Auburn University, an M.S. in 1983 at the Louisiana State University School of Medicine, and a Ph.D. in 1987 at the University of Florida. He was a post-doctoral fellow and associate research scientist at the Yale University School of Medicine from 1987 to 1991. In 1991, he joined the U.S. Centers for Disease Control and Prevention's (CDC's) Division of Parasitic Diseases, where he served as chief of the Vector Genetics Section from 1999 to 2003. In 2003 he moved to CDC's Division of Vector-Borne Diseases in Fort Collins, Colorado, to become chief of the Bacterial Diseases Branch. In this capacity, he coordinated CDC's programs on Lyme borreliosis, tick-borne relapsing fever, Bartonella, plague, and tularemia. During his tenure at CDC, Dr. Beard has worked in the prevention of vector-borne diseases, in both the domestic and the global arenas. In addition to his work as chief of the Bacterial Diseases Branch, from 2011 until 2017 Dr. Beard served as the associate director for climate change in CDC's National Center for Emerging and Zoonotic Infectious Diseases, where he coordinated CDC's efforts to mitigate the potential impact of climate variability and disruption on infectious diseases in humans. In this capacity he participated in the U.S. Global Change Research Program Climate Change and Human Health Group and was an editor and lead author on the 2016 report, *The Impacts of Climate Change on Human Health in the United States: A Scientific Assessment*. In 2017, he was appointed as the deputy director of CDC's Division of Vector-Borne Diseases. He has published more than 140 scientific papers, books, and book chapters collectively, and has served on a variety of committees and panels both inside and outside CDC, including working groups or advisory panels for the World Health Organization, the Bill & Melinda Gates Foundation, and the American Meteorological Society. He is an associate editor for *Emerging Infectious Diseases* and past president of the Society for Vector Ecology and served as deputy incident manager for CDC's Zika virus outbreak response. He also served as associate director for science for task forces in CDC's 2014 Ebola response and currently in CDC's COVID-19 response. Beard has served as CDC's representative to the U.S. Department of Health and Human Services Tick-Borne Disease Working Group federal advisory committee since its establishment in 2017.

Christopher Braden, M.D., serves as the deputy director, National Center for Emerging and Zoonotic Infectious Diseases at the U.S. Centers for Disease Control and Prevention (CDC). Prior to 2016, he was the director of the Division of Foodborne, Waterborne and Environmental Diseases. Previously, he served as the associate director for science in the Division of Parasitic Diseases, and chief of outbreak response and surveillance in the Division of Foodborne, Bacterial and Mycotic Diseases. Dr. Braden has served on incident management teams for multiple national and international CDC responses.

Dr. Braden received his bachelor of science from Cornell University, and his M.D. at the University of New Mexico School of Medicine. He completed his internship and residency in internal medicine and then his fellowship in infectious diseases at Tufts New England Medical Center in Boston, Massachusetts. He is board certified in infectious diseases. He joined CDC as an Epidemic Intelligence Service officer in 1993. He is a retired commissioned officer in the U.S. Public Health Service, and a member of the Infectious Diseases Society of America.

He has authored more than 70 peer-reviewed publications and textbook chapters. His major areas of interest include molecular epidemiology of infectious diseases, infectious diseases surveillance and outbreak investigation, and national programs in food safety.

Carlos das Neves D.V.M., Ph.D., Dipl.ECZM, graduated in veterinary medicine, from the Technical University of Lisbon in 2004, and obtained his doctorate (Ph.D.) in veterinary science, specialty virology in 2009 from the Norwegian School of Veterinary Science. With scientific papers published in international scientific journals and extensive experience in scientific project coordination Dr. das Neves is currently the director of research and internationalization at the Norwegian Veterinary Institute in Oslo, responsible for coordination of a research staff of more than 150 researchers working in more than 20 different disciplines. He served previously for 3 years as head of virology and 2 years as head of food safety and emerging threats at the Norwegian Veterinary Institute. He holds a joint position at the Faculty of Medical Sciences at the University of Tromsø, and was promoted to research professor in 2018. Dr. das Neves has developed his scientific research in the field of virology in wildlife species and has done extensive fieldwork across the Arctic region. He now works with topics related to One Health and emerging threats, especially viral zoonosis and antimicrobial resistance, with a focus on low- and middle-income countries. In 2013 he earned the diploma of specialist in wildlife population health at the European College of Zoological Medicine and was appointed by the Norwegian Government in 2014 as an expert in animal welfare and health of the National Food Safety Committee. He is currently the president of the Wildlife Disease Association, the Wildlife Population Health specialty chair for the European College of Zoological Medicine, and member of the IUCN Species Survival Commission–Wildlife Health Specialist Group. In 2020, Norway appointed Dr. das Neves to the group of international experts at the Intergovernmental Science-Policy Platform on Biodiversity and Ecosystem Services working on the relationships between biodiversity and pandemics. He is also a commissioner at the Lancet One Health Commission, and a member of the Lancet COVID-19 Commission Task Force.

Peter Daszak, Ph.D., is president of EcoHealth Alliance, a U.S.-based organization that conducts research and outreach programs on global health, conservation, and international development. Dr. Daszak's research has been instrumental in identifying and predicting the impacts of emerging diseases across the globe. His achievements include identifying the bat origin of severe acute respiratory syndrome, identifying the underlying drivers of Nipah and Hendra virus emergence, producing the first ever global emerging disease hot spots map, developing a strategy to find out how many unknown viruses exist that could threaten to become pandemic, identifying the first case of a species extinction due to disease, and discovering the disease chytridiomycosis as the cause of global amphibian declines. Dr. Daszak is a member and chair of the National Academies of Sciences, Engineering and Medicine's Forum on Microbial Threats. He is a member of the National Research Council (NRC) Advisory Committee to the U.S. Global Change Research Program, the Supervisory Board of the One Health Platform, the One Health Commission Council of Advisors, the Center of Excellence for Emerging and Zoonotic Animal Diseases External Advisory Board, the Cosmos Club, and the Advisory Council of the Bridge Collaborative; he has served on the Institute of Medicine committee on global surveillance for emerging zoonoses, the NRC committee on the future of veterinary research, and the International Standing Advisory Board of the Australian Biosecurity Cooperative Research Centres, and has advised the Director for Medical Preparedness Policy on the White House National Security Staff on global health issues. Dr. Daszak is a regular advisor to the World Health Organization (WHO), World Organisation for Animal Health, and the Food and Agriculture Organization of the United Nations, and is actively involved in the WHO Expert group on Public Health Emergency Disease Prioritization. Dr. Daszak won the 2000 Commonwealth

Scientific and Industrial Research Organisation medal for collaborative research on the discovery of amphibian chytridiomycosis, is the EHA institutional lead for the U.S. Agency for International Development–Emerging Pandemic Threats–PREDICT, is on the editorial boards of *Conservation Biology*, *One Health*, and *Transactions of the Royal Society of Tropical Medicine & Hygiene*, and is editor-in-chief of the journal *EcoHealth*. He has authored more than 300 scientific papers, and his work has been the focus of extensive media coverage, ranging from popular press articles to television appearances.

Victor del Rio Vilas, D.V.M., M.Sc., M.B.A., Ph.D., is currently at the World Health Organization (WHO), South East Asia Regional Office in New Delhi, India, where he coordinates the Global Outbreak Alert and Response Network in the region. He was previously at the Department of Epidemiology, School of Veterinary Medicine, University of Surrey (UK), and at the Centre on Global Health Security at Chatham House, London. Until January 2018 he worked at WHO-Geneva on the development of WHO's epidemic vulnerability evaluation framework. Until November 2016, Dr. Del Rio was a consultant with the Pan American Health Organization (PAHO/WHO), based in Rio de Janeiro, Brazil. In that capacity, Dr. Del Rio advised ministries/departments of health across the PAHO region on epidemiology, surveillance, and control measures for a number of diseases, such as rabies, leishmaniasis, echinococcosis, and yellow fever and on zoonoses programmatic issues. He also contributed to WHO's global response to the Ebola virus disease outbreak in Liberia in 2015, previously worked in Uzbekistan implementing the Biological Threat Reduction Program (Defence Threat Reduction Agency, U.S. Department of Defense), and served as veterinary advisor and epidemiologist for United Kingdom's Department for Environment, Food and Rural Affairs (Defra), and the Veterinary Laboratories Agency.

Kaylee Myhre Errecaborde, D.V.M., Ph.D., is a policy researcher and a veterinarian. Kaylee supports health workers to situate their technical work within the context of international policies and frameworks. As a technical consultant at World Health Organization headquarters in Geneva, Switzerland, she works on the Human and Animal Interface Team, supporting member countries to build capacity for collaborative, One Health preparedness and response for zoonotic disease. As faculty at the University of Minnesota, her research focuses on global approaches to health workforce development, collaborative governance, policy, and international trade capacity. She previously worked for the U.S. Congress on global health, border health, international trade, and food security issues with the U.S. House Foreign Affairs Committee and later on the U.S. Senate Homeland Security Committee.

Julie Fischer, Ph.D., is a senior technical advisor for global health at Civilian Research and Development Foundation (CRDF) Global, where she is the primary investigator on several projects that aim to strengthen capacities to prevent, detect, and respond to emerging disease threats in South and Southeast Asia, Central Asia, and the Middle East and North Africa. Prior to joining CRDF, she served as an associate research professor in the Department of Microbiology and Immunology and director of the Elizabeth R. Griffin Program at Georgetown University, where she led a multidisciplinary team to promote evidence-based biosafety and biosecurity practices, and to help partner nations strengthen their capacities to detect and characterize disease threats rapidly, reliably, accurately, and safely. Before she joined Georgetown, Dr. Fischer held leadership positions at George Washington University's Milken Institute School of Public Health and the Global Health Security Program at the Stimson Center. Dr. Fischer received a B.A. from Hollins University, and a Ph.D. in microbiology and immunology from Vanderbilt University, and completed post-doctoral training in viral pathogenesis at the University of Washington and Seattle Biomedical Research Institute.

Greg Glass, Ph.D., is a professor in the Department of Geography and the Emerging Pathogens Institute at the University of Florida, Gainesville (UF). He received his Ph.D. in population biology/quantitative methods at the University of Kansas and his post-doctoral fellowship in the Department of Immunology & Infectious Diseases at the Johns Hopkins School of Public Health, where he worked on characterizing the transmission systems and health consequences of hantaviruses. The group was responsible for establishing the tight associations of reservoir species and viruses, as well as developing diagnostic methods and performing human population surveys of viral spillover. He remained at Johns Hopkins University with faculty appointments in the Departments of Molecular Microbiology and Immunology and Epidemiology studying vector-borne and zoonotic agents for 30 years before moving to UF, where he has continued developing applications for detailed characterizations of space–time dynamics of these disease systems in the environment. He has served on numerous national and international committees for the National Aeronautics and Space Administration, the National Institutes of Health, the National Academy of Sciences, the World Health Organization, and the U.S. Centers for Disease Control and Prevention. During the past decade much of his effort has focused in Eastern Europe and South Asia providing training on pathogen detection and surveillance.

David Goldman, M.D., M.P.H., joined the U.S. Food and Drug Administration's Office of Food Policy and Response as chief medical officer effective January 15, 2019.

Dr. Goldman provides medical and scientific leadership to the foods program and provides strategic guidance on medical and public health issues associated with food, dietary supplements, cosmetic products, and the nutritional composition of food. He is a clinical expert on issues related to food safety and a key leader in helping the agency respond to food safety outbreak and recall events.

As chief medical officer for the foods program, Dr. Goldman plays a pivotal role in continuing to advance the agency's work to improve our recall efforts by co-chairing the Strategic Coordinated Oversight of Recall Execution team. Dr. Goldman's work also includes the full portfolio of work previously led by the Center for Food Safety and Applied Nutrition's (CFSAN) chief medical officer. This includes providing leadership to foods program medical officers and chairing CFSAN's Health Hazard Evaluation Board, which evaluates the human health effects of physical, microbiological, chemical, or radiological contamination of food and cosmetic products. Dr. Goldman also serves as a spokesperson on human health issues associated with food products, involving food safety, nutrition, and cosmetics. In addition, he serves as liaison to the U.S. Department of Agriculture (USDA) in foodborne outbreak situations.

Dr. Goldman has considerable experience in issues directly relevant to these important roles. He most recently served as the chief medical officer of the Food Safety and Inspection Service (FSIS), which is part of the USDA. In this role, he was responsible for occupational health issues related to chemical and biological exposures, as well as providing medical expertise on emerging food safety issues. He was assistant administrator for FSIS's Office of Public Health Science from November 2004 through May 2018, leading a staff of 300 that provided the scientific foundation for FSIS policies, conducted microbial risk assessments, and executed a national sampling program of meat and poultry products. In addition, at the appointment of the U.S. surgeon general, Dr. Goldman served as the U.S. Public Health Service (USPHS) chief professional officer for physicians from 2013 to 2017.

Dr. Goldman is a board-certified family medicine and preventive medicine/public health physician and a member of the Commissioned Corps of the U.S. Public Health Service since February 2002. He spent 10 years in the U.S. Army Medical Corps, practicing both family medicine and preventive medicine. He then spent 3½ years at the Virginia Department of Health, first as a district health director, then briefly as the deputy state epidemiologist, before joining the USPHS and FSIS. Dr. Goldman received his bachelor of arts from the University of Virginia, and his doctor of medicine from the University of Virginia. He holds a master of public health in epidemiology from the University of Washington.

Eric Goosby, M.D., is an internationally recognized expert on infectious diseases, with a specialty in HIV/AIDS clinical care, research, and policy. During the Clinton administration, Dr. Goosby was the founding director of the Ryan White CARE Act, the largest federally funded HIV/AIDS program in the United States. He went on to become the interim director of the White House's Office of National AIDS Policy. In the Obama administration, Dr. Goosby was appointed ambassador-at-large and implemented the U.S. President's Emergency Plan for AIDS Relief (PEPFAR), which significantly expanded under his tenure life-saving HIV treatment to millions in sub-Saharan Africa, Southeast Asia, and Eastern Europe.

After serving as the U.S. global AIDS coordinator, he was appointed by the UN secretary-general as the special envoy for TB (tuberculosis), where he focused on the first-ever UN High-Level Meeting on TB in 2019. He is currently a professor of medicine at the University of California, San Francisco, School of Medicine, and leading the Center for Global Health Delivery, Diplomacy and Economics, Institute for Global Health Sciences. He is also a member of the Biden COVID-19 Advisory Board, a member of the Western States Scientific Safety Review Workgroup, and serves on the San Francisco Department of Public Health Policy Group for the COVID-19 Response.

Barbara Han, Ph.D., is a disease ecologist at the Cary Institute of Ecosystem Studies. Her research program builds predictive capacity for zoonotic diseases that aim to better target upstream surveillance and management activities to preempt spillover transmission to humans. She has pioneered the application of machine learning and ecoinformatics approaches to predict zoonotic animal hosts and insect vectors, with recent work incorporating these approaches with mathematical modeling and structural modeling to quantify spillover risks posed by multiple animal species to humans (e.g., severe acute respiratory syndrome coronavirus 2). This work continues to inform the creation of new research and policy initiatives at the intersection of artificial intelligence, disease ecology, biodefense, biomedical science, and global health. She currently serves as the principal investigator (PI) or co-PI on multi-institution and multinational grants funded by the National Science Foundation, the National Institutes of Health, and the Defense Advanced Research Projects Agency.

Eva Harris, Ph.D., is a professor in the Division of Infectious Diseases in the School of Public Health and director of the Center for Global Public Health at the University of California, Berkeley. She has developed a multidisciplinary approach to study the molecular virology, pathogenesis, immunology, epidemiology, clinical aspects, and control of dengue, Zika, and chikungunya, the most prevalent mosquito-borne viral diseases in humans. Specifially, her work addresses immune correlates of protection and pathogenesis, viral and host factors that modulate disease severity, and virus replication and evolution, using in vitro approaches, animal models, and research involving human populations. This has been possible through a close collaboration with the Ministry of Health in Nicaragua for more than 28 years. Her international work focuses on laboratory-based and epidemiological studies of dengue, chikungunya, Zika, and influenza in endemic Latin American countries, particularly in Nicaragua, where ongoing projects include clinical and biological studies of severe dengue, a pediatric cohort study of dengue, Zika, chikungunya, and influenza transmission in Managua, a household transmission study of Zika, and a recently concluded cluster-randomized controlled trial of evidence-based, community-derived interventions for prevention of dengue via control of its mosquito vector. She is also directing a study of Zika in infants and pregnancy in Nicaragua and evaluating a number of Zika diagnostic tests with her team in Nicaragua. In 1997, she received a MacArthur Award for work over the previous 10 years developing programs to build scientific capacity in developing countries to address public health and infectious disease issues. This enabled her to found a nonprofit organization in 1998, Sustainable Sciences Institute (SSI; www.sustainablesciences.org), with offices in San Francisco, Nicaragua, and Egypt, to continue and expand this work. Dr. Harris was named a Pew Scholar for her work on dengue pathogenesis. She received a national recognition award from the minister of health of Nicaragua for her contribution to scientific development and was selected as a "Global Leader for Tomorrow" by the World Economic Forum. In 2012, she was elected councilor of the American Society of Tropical Medicine and Hygiene and received a Global Citizen Award from the United Nations Association. She has published more than 200 peer-reviewed articles, as well as a book on her international scientific work.

James Hospedales, M.D., M.Sc., is founder of the EarthMedic and EarthNurse Foundation for Planetary Health, which aims to mobilize health professionals concerned about the climate and health crisis to take action to improve health of self, society, and planet. Dr. Hospedales also serves as chair of the Defeat-NCD Partnership, aiming to address noncommunicable diseases in low- and middle-income countries. He served as inaugural executive director, Caribbean Public Health Agency, 2013–2019, serving 23 countries, in which role he chaired an expert panel on climate change and health in the Caribbean. Previously, Dr. Hospedales was senior advisor and coordinator for Prevention and Control of Chronic Diseases, Pan American Health Organization/World Health Organization. From 1998 to 2006, Dr. Hospedales was the director of the Caribbean Epidemiology Centre, serving 21 countries. He played a key role in developing partnerships for HIV/AIDS prevention, and for improving health, safety, and environmental conditions in the Caribbean travel and tourism industry. Dr. Hospedales was a member of the Caribbean Commission on Health and Development, which made policy recommendations to the heads of government and named chronic diseases as a super-priority for the region. This work helped stimulate the UN high-level meetings on noncommunicable diseases in 2011, 2014 and 2018. Dr. Hospedales's career has included service as an epidemic intelligence service officer with the U.S. Centers for Disease Control and Prevention, as an epidemiologist at the Caribbean Epidemiology Centre, and several years working in public health for the UK National Health Service. Dr. Hospedales graduated with honors in medicine from University of the West Indies in 1980. He has an M.Sc. in community medicine from the London School of Hygiene & Tropical Medicine, is a fellow of the UK Faculty of Public Health, and an accredited partnership broker with The Partnering Institute (TPI). He has published more than 100 papers and reports.

Kate Huebner, V.M.D., M.S., is a veterinary medical officer within the Office of Surveillance and Compliance at the U.S. Food and Drug Administration's Center for Veterinary Medicine. Dr. Huebner obtained her veterinary degree from the University of Pennsylvania and went on to complete an internship in livestock medicine and surgery at Colorado State University (CSU). She also obtained her master's in clinical sciences at CSU, researching the effects of a feed additive on feedlot cattle liver abscess prevalence, fecal microbiomes, and antimicrobial resistance. Dr. Huebner enjoys working on regulatory and policy matters related to innovative science and technologies affecting human, animal, and environmental health.

Olga B. Jonas is an economist and a senior fellow at the Harvard Global Health Institute, after serving as an economist at the World Bank in 1983–2016. She coordinated the World Bank's operational responses to avian flu and pandemics in 2005–2013 and implementation of reforms of emergency response financing policies. Jointly with the United Nations system influenza coordinator, David Nabarro, she was the lead World Bank author of five global monitoring reports on country and global programs in 2005–2010 that saw increased use of One Health approaches for prevention and preparedness in nearly 100 developing countries, helped by $3.9 billion of external financing.

She was also lead author of the World Bank's 2016 report on antimicrobial resistance, the parts on pandemics in the World Bank's *2014 World Development Report on Risks to Development*, and the economic analysis in the *2012 Economics of One Health* report; she co-authored *International Cooperative Responses to Pandemic Threats: A Critical Analysis* (2015).

Earlier she worked as a macroeconomist for policy-reform programs in Africa and Asia and then as financing and development policy adviser for two replenishments of the International Development Association (the World Bank's fund for the poorest countries), small states task force, fragile states, and responses to major disasters.

She now focuses on pandemic and epidemic risks through understanding of links to economic development, governance to increase the adequacy and effectiveness of financing of prevention, preparedness and responses to microbial threats, policies to contain antimicrobial resistance, and the role of One Health approaches.

Laura Kahn, M.D., M.P.H., is a physician and research scholar with the Program on Science and Global Security at the Princeton University School of Public and International Affairs. In 2006, she published "Confronting Zoonoses, Linking Human and Veterinary Medicine" in the CDC journal *Emerging Infectious Diseases*, which helped launch the One Health Initiative (http://www.onehealthinitiative.com), a global effort to promote the One Health concept that human, animal, and environmental/ecosystem health are linked. She is the author of two books: *Who's in Charge? Leadership During Epidemics, Bioterror Attacks, and Other Public Health Crises* (2nd edition published in 2020) and *One Health and the Politics of Antimicrobial Resistance* (2016). In June 2020, she launched her Coursera course: Bats, Ducks, and Pandemics: An Introduction to One Health Policy, which has more than 4,000 students enrolled from around the world. In 2014, she received a Presidential Award for Meritorious Service from the American Association of Public Health Physicians, and in 2016, the American Veterinary Epidemiology Society awarded her with their highest honor for her work in One Health: the K.F. Meyer-James H. Steele Gold Head Cane Award.

Esron Karimuribo, B.V.M., M.V.M., Ph.D., is a One Health epidemiology professor and director of Postgraduate Studies and Research at Sokoine University of Agriculture (SUA) based in Morogoro, Tanzania. He also works with the Southern African Centre for Infectious Disease Surveillance (SACIDS) Foundation for One Health, a regional disease surveillance network which is headquartered at SUA. Dr. Karimuribo holds BVM and MVM degrees from SUA and a Ph.D. from the University of Reading in the United Kingdom.

In 2009, Dr. Karimuribo joined SACIDS as a postdoctoral research fellow working on resource mapping and application of mobile technologies in infectious disease surveillance. Through the financial support from the Skoll Global Threats Fund/Ending Pandemics, Dr. Karimuribo led a team that designed and developed an app called AfyaData, which has been rolled out to support disease surveillance in human and animal health sectors in East and southern African countries. On July 1, 2019, the AfyaData team was awarded a prize by the Fondation Pierre Fabre. Dr. Karimuribo has published more than 100 articles in peer-reviewed international journals. He is a member of various professional associations and communities within and outside Tanzania.

Kent E. Kester, M.D., is currently vice president and head of Translational Science and Biomarkers at Sanofi Pasteur. During a 24-year career in the U.S. Army, he worked extensively in clinical vaccine development and led multiple research platforms at the Walter Reed Army Institute of Research, the U.S. Department of Defense's largest and most diverse biomedical research laboratory—an institution he later led as its commander/director. His final military assignment was as the associate dean for clinical research in the School of Medicine at the Uniformed Services University of the Health Sciences (USUHS). Dr. Kester holds an undergraduate degree from Bucknell University and an M.D. from Jefferson Medical College. He completed his internship and residency in internal medicine at the University of Maryland and a fellowship in infectious diseases at the Walter Reed Army Medical Center. A malaria vaccine researcher with more than 70 scientific manuscripts and book chapters, Dr. Kester has played a major role in the development of the malaria vaccine candidate known as RTS,S. Currently a member of the Presidential Advisory Council on Combating Antibiotic-Resistant Bacteria, he previously chaired the steering committee of the National Institute of Allergy and Infectious Diseases (NIAID)-USUHS Infectious Disease Clinical Research Program, and has served as a member of the Food and Drug Administration's Vaccines and Related Biologics Products Advisory Committee, the NIAID Advisory Council, and the U.S. Centers for Disease Control and Prevention's Office of Infectious Diseases Board of Scientific Counselors. Board certified in both internal medicine and infectious diseases, he holds faculty appointments at USUHS and the University of Maryland, and is a fellow of the American College of Physicians, the Infectious Diseases Society of America, and the American Society of Tropical Medicine and Hygiene.

Lonnie King, D.V.M., M.S., M.P.A., A.C.V.P.M., has served as dean for three colleges over 17 years. Most recently, he was the interim dean of the College of Food, Agricultural and Environmental Sciences at The Ohio State University and was also the vice president for agriculture. He was also dean of the College of Veterinary Medicine at The Ohio State University from 2009 to 2015. At Ohio State, Dr. King held the Ruth Stanton Endowed Chair and served as the executive dean for the seven health science colleges at the university. Before becoming dean at OSU, he was the first director of the National Center for Zoonotic, Vector-Borne, and Enteric Diseases at the

U.S. Centers for Disease Control and Prevention. Dr. King led the center's activities for surveillance, diagnostics, disease investigations, epidemiology, research, public education, policy development, and disease prevention and public health concerns. Before serving as director, he was the first chief of the agency's Office of Strategy and Innovation.

Dr. King served as dean of the College of Veterinary Medicine, Michigan State University, from 1996 to 2006. He led the college's academic programs, research, the teaching hospital, the diagnostic center for population and animal health, basic and clinical science departments, and the outreach and continuing education programs. He was also professor of large animal clinical sciences and a distinguished university professor.

In 1992, Dr. King was appointed administrator for the Animal and Plant Health Inspection Service (APHIS), U.S. Department of Agriculture (USDA), in Washington, DC. In this role, he provided executive leadership and direction for ensuring the health and care of animals and plants, to improve agricultural productivity and competitiveness, and to contribute to the national economy and public health. Dr. King also served as the country's chief veterinary officer for five years and worked extensively in global trade and closely with the World Organisation for Animal Health (OIE). He also served as the deputy administrator for Veterinary Services of APHIS, USDA, where he led national efforts in disease eradication, imports and exports, diagnostic labs, and animal welfare.

As a native of Wooster, Ohio, Dr. King received his B.S. and D.V.M. degrees from The Ohio State University. He earned his M.S. in epidemiology from the University of Minnesota and received his master's degree in public administration from the American University. Dr. King is a board-certified member of the American College of Veterinary Preventive Medicine and has completed the Senior Executive Fellowship program at Harvard University. Dr. King was elected as a member of the National Academy of Medicine in 2004. He is a past vice-chair of the National Academies of Sciences, Engineering, and Medicine's Forum on Microbial Threats to Health and has been awarded both the Global One Health Award presented in 2013 by the World Small Animal Veterinary Medical Association and the OIE Meritorious Award for his distinguished global career in animal and public health in 2019. His interests and expertise are in emerging zoonoses, antimicrobial resistance, global health, One Health, and leadership development. He is currently the vice-chair for the Presidential Advisory Council Combating Antibiotic-Resistant Bacteria and is serving on the boards or in advisory roles for 10 organizations and companies.

Andrew Maccabe, D.V.M., M.P.H., J.D., is the chief executive officer of the Association of American Veterinary Medical Colleges (AAVMC). He received his bachelor of science and doctor of veterinary medicine degrees from The Ohio State University in 1981 and 1985, respectively. Dr. Maccabe began his professional career in Jefferson, Ohio, where he worked in a mixed animal practice with primary emphasis on dairy herd health.

In 1988, he was commissioned as a public health officer in the U.S. Air Force, where he managed the preventive medicine activities of several Air Force installations and directed programs in occupational health, communicable disease control, and health promotion.

Dr. Maccabe completed his master of public health degree at Harvard University in 1995. That same year he became chief of the Health Risk Assessment Branch of the U.S. Air Force, where he directed the health risk assessment program for environmental restoration activities throughout the Air Force.

Dr. Maccabe completed his juris doctor degree, magna cum laude, at the University of Arizona in 2002. He subsequently became the associate executive director at AAVMC, where he led programs to advance veterinary medical education. In 2007, he was appointed as the U.S. Centers for Disease Control and Prevention's liaison to the U.S. Food and Drug Administration, where he coordinated policies and programs between the two agencies before returning to AAVMC in 2012 as the CEO.

Dr. Maccabe holds memberships in many professional organizations, including the American Veterinary Medical Association, the District of Columbia Veterinary Medical Association, and the Pride Veterinary Medical Community. He is a member of the State Bar of Arizona, the Bar of the District of Columbia, and a licensed patent attorney. After 24 years of service in the U.S. Air Force, he retired as a colonel in 2017.

Catherine Machalaba, Ph.D., serves as senior policy advisor and a senior scientist at EcoHealth Alliance, a scientific non-profit organization working at the nexus of conservation, global health, and capacity strengthening. Her work focuses on assessing and optimizing One Health strategies, including the use of economic analyses to identify cost-effective options to reduce the threat and impact of emerging infectious diseases. She was a lead author of the World Bank Operational Framework for Strengthening Human, Animal and Environmental Public Health Systems at their Interface ("One Health Operational Framework") published in 2018 to assist countries and donor institutions in implementing One Health approaches. Dr. Machalaba is the program officer for the International Union for the Conservation of Nature Species Survival Commission Wildlife Health Specialist Group, and previously served as chair of the American Public Health Association (APHA) Veterinary Public Health group, where she led development of APHA's One Health policy statement. She holds degrees in biology and public health and a Ph.D. in environmental and planetary health sciences.

Jonna Mazet, D.V.M., M.P.V.M., Ph.D. (*Co-Chair*), earned her doctorate of veterinary medicine, master of preventive medicine, and Ph.D. in epidemiology from the University of California, Davis (UC Davis). In addition to her faculty appointment in the Department of Medicine and Epidemiology in the UC Davis School of Veterinary Medicine, she serves as the executive director of the UC Davis One Health Institute (OHI). Dr. Mazet specializes in emerging infectious diseases and wildlife epidemiology, and as director of OHI, focuses on global health problem solving. In her role at UC Davis, she assists government agencies and the public with emerging health challenges and is active in international One Health research programs, such as tuberculosis in Africa, novel pathogen detection in less developed countries, and pathogen pollution of California coastal waters. Dr. Mazet founded California's Oiled Wildlife Care Network, the premier model wildlife emergency management system worldwide, and remains a consulting expert on wildlife emergency preparedness and response, serving on multiple governmental and nongovernmental organization (NGO) advisory panels. Dr. Mazet is the principal investigator and global director of the novel viral emergence early warning project, PREDICT, that has been developed with the U.S. Agency for International Development's Emerging Pandemic Threats Program. She leads a network of global NGOs and governmental agencies to build capacity within the PREDICT-engaged countries to develop surveillance systems and complete the necessary research to halt the next pandemic, like influenza, severe acute respiratory syndrome, Ebola, and HIV that have preceded the program.

Tracey McNamara, D.V.M., Diplomate, A.C.V.P., is a veterinary pathologist and a professor of pathology at Western University of Health Sciences College of Veterinary Medicine in Pomona, California. Dr. McNamara specializes in the recognition and understanding of the diseases of captive and free-ranging wildlife and is best known for her work on the discovery of the West Nile virus in 1999. In 2004 she worked on the Defense Threat Reduction Agency's Integrated Biosurveillance for Zoonotic Threats program in Uzbekistan, Kazakhstan, and Georgia. She served as lead on a project with Russian colleagues on the "Human–Animal Interface: Improving Biological Threat Detection and Surveillance in Russia" by the Nuclear Threat Initiative's Global Health and Biosecurity program in Washington, DC. Dr. McNamara served as a consultant to the National Biosurveillance Advisory Subcommittee from 2008 to 2009 and continues to be actively involved in the development of the nation's biosurveillance strategy. She recently gave a TEDxUCLA talk entitled "Canaries in the Coalmine" about continued gaps in biosurveillance for emerging biological threats. Dr. McNamara is a founding member of the Global Health Security Alliance working with German/U.S. military, the United Nations, medical intelligence, and security sectors. She chaired a panel on "Disease X" at the World Health Summit, Berlin, 2018. She helped organize a meeting at the Salzburg Global Seminar on One Health Metrics in November 2019 and is a Salzburg fellow. She is actively involved in the One Health movement and advocates for a species-neutral approach to the detection of pandemic threats. Most recently, she was asked to be a member of the Red Dawn Breaking Team on COVID-19, a group of experts advising the assistant secretary for preparedness and response of the United States.

Carrie S. McNeil, D.V.M., M.P.H., is a veterinary epidemiologist at Sandia National Laboratories with a background in public policy and emergency management who has designed numerous strategic and operational-level exercises and drills to evaluate One Health preparedness in North Africa, the Middle East, and South and Southeast Asia. She coauthored Portal for Readiness Exercises and Planning (PREP), a no-cost, web-based platform tracking multiplayer, role-based, participant-led exercises and planning workshops. On behalf of Ending Pandemics, Dr. McNeil and her team have designed and are implementing a series of During Action Reviews for COVID-19 at national and subnational levels internationally. She has led multiyear One Health Biothreat Readiness Leadership trainings globally using PREP. She is principal investigator on a One Health–focused assessment of domestic Food–Agriculture–Veterinary readiness on behalf of the U.S. Department of Homeland Security and on research leveraging remote technologies and machine learning for early outbreak detection. Prior to coming to Sandia, she served as an Epidemic Intelligence Service officer for the U.S. Centers for Disease Control and Prevention and as an emergency response planner with the CDC. She received an M.P.H. with honors in global environmental health at Rollins School of Public Health, where she conducted a participatory-based community health assessment in one of the country's most rural and impoverished counties. As a former committee consultant with the California State Legislature and director of a water-quality nonprofit, she worked to ensure that science was incorporated in developing health, environment, and preparedness policies. After completing her D.V.M. at the University of California, Davis, in 2004 and an internship in 2006, Dr. McNeil practiced in small animal emergency medicine and became a veterinary medical officer with the National Veterinary Response Team.

John Nkengasong, M.Sc., Ph.D., currently serves as director of the Africa Centres for Disease Control and Prevention, a specialized technical institution of the African Union.

In early 2020, he was appointed as one of the World Health Organization director-general's special envoys on COVID-19 preparedness and response. In addition, Dr. Nkengasong was most recently awarded the Bill & Melinda Gates Foundation's 2020 Global Goalkeeper Award for his contributions to the continental response in fighting the COVID-19 pandemic in Africa.

Prior to his current position, he served as acting deputy principal director of the Center for Global Health and chief of the International Laboratory Branch, Division of Global HIV and tuberculosis for the U.S. Centers for Disease Control and Prevention (CDC).

Dr. Nkengasong holds a master's degree in tropical biomedical science from the Institute of Tropical Medicine in Antwerp, Belgium, and a doctorate in medical sciences (virology) from the University of Brussels, Belgium.

Dr. Nkengasong has received numerous awards for his work including the Sheppard Award and the William Watson Medal of Excellence, the highest recognition awarded by CDC. He is also a recipient of the Knight of Honour Medal from the Government of Cote d'Ivoire, was knighted in 2017 as the officer of Loin by the president of Senegal, H.E. Macky Sall, and knighted in November 2018 by the government of Cameroon for his significant contributions to public health. He is an adjunct professor at the Emory School of Public Health, Emory University, Atlanta, Georgia.

He serves on several international advisory boards, including the Coalition for Epidemic Preparedness Initiative and the International AIDS Vaccine Initiative, among others. He has authored more than 250 peer-reviewed articles in international journals and published several book chapters.

Thierry Nyatanyi, M.D., M.P.H., M.M.Sc., is a physician by training and a global health specialist. Previously, Nyatanyi worked with the Ministry of Health in Rwanda, and with the University of Minnesota in the United States. In Rwanda, he served as the director of the epidemiology department, and head of the division for epidemic surveillance and response at the Ministry of Health. In that capacity, he was responsible for developing and implementing programs meant to prevent and rapidly respond to emerging and re-emerging infectious disease threats. In the United States, he has worked with the University of Minnesota as the regional technical lead for Africa, under the U.S. Agency for International Development (USAID)-funded One Health Workforce Project that supported higher institutions of learning (public health and veterinary medicine) to develop a public health workforce with the technical skills and cross-sectoral capacity to readily adapt and respond to emerging infectious disease threats in eight African countries. He has also worked as an international consultant with the Food and Agriculture Organization of the United Nations to assess One Health operationalization gaps in the Africa region. He also served as the senior advisor on the COVID-19 response with the Africa Centres for Disease Control and Prevention, supporting the Ministry of Health in Rwanda.

Currently, he is working with the USAID mission in Ivory Coast as the Global Health Security Agenda senior consultant. He is fluent in English and French. He received an M.D./M.P.H from the University of Rwanda, and an M.M.Sc. in global health delivery from Harvard Medical School.

Jonathan ("Jono") D. Quick, M.D., M.P.H., is an internationally known global health leader and the author of *The End of Epidemics: The Looming Threat to Humanity and How to Stop It* (www.endofepidemics.com 2018, 2020). Drawing lessons from the last 100 years on how to prevent epidemics from spreading worldwide, Dr. Quick has been interviewed about the COVID-19 pandemic by North American, European, and Asian media. A family physician and health management specialist, Dr. Quick is managing director for Pandemic Response, Preparedness, and Prevention at The Rockefeller Foundation and adjunct professor of global health at the Duke Global Health Institute. He has served as president and chief executive officer of the global health nonprofit Management Sciences for Health, director of essential medicines at the World Health Organization, and resident advisor for health system development and financing programs in Afghanistan and Kenya. Dr. Quick has carried out assignments to improve the health and lives of people in more than 70 countries in Africa, Asia, Latin America, and the Middle East. He also holds faculty appointments at Harvard Medical School and the University of Boston School of Public Health; is a past fellow of the Royal Society of Medicine; and has a first degree from Harvard University and an M.D., with distinction in research, and master of public health from the University of Rochester.

Peter Rabinowitz, M.D., M.P.H., is a board-certified physician and a Professor at the University of Washington (UW), jointly appointed in environmental and occupational health sciences, global health, and family medicine, with adjunct appointments in the Department of Medicine Division of Allergy and Infectious Disease as well as the Department of Epidemiology. He has more than 20 years of research experience with a current focus on zoonotic diseases, and more than 100 publications and 20 book chapters on zoonotic and emerging infectious diseases, One Health, and occupational medicine. He is the director of the Center for One Health Research at UW that focuses on zoonotic diseases and other health connections between humans, animals, and environments. He has a particular interest in increasing the involvement of human health professionals in One Health research and practice related to zoonotic diseases.

David Rizzo, Ph.D., received his doctorate in plant pathology from the University of Minnesota and subsequently joined the faculty of the University of California, Davis, Department of Plant Pathology and the Graduate

Group in Ecology in 1995. In 2013, Dr. Rizzo became chair of the Department of Plant Pathology. Research in his lab focuses on the ecology and management of tree diseases, including diseases caused by both native and introduced pathogens. Research in the lab takes a multi-scale approach ranging from experimental studies on the basic biology of organisms to field studies across landscapes. In addition to research, Dr. Rizzo teaches a number of courses in One Health and mycology. He is director of the One Health–focused undergraduate major, global disease biology. The major is a collaboration between the Department of Plant Pathology in the College of Agricultural and Environmental Sciences, the School of Veterinary Medicine, and the School of Medicine at UC Davis. Since 2004, he has also been director of the Science and Society program in the College of Agricultural and Environmental Sciences. Science and Society is an academic program designed to offer students the opportunity to discover the interdisciplinary connections that link the biological, physical, and social sciences with societal issues and cultural discourses.

Cristina Romanelli, M.A., M.Sc., is the interagency liaison for the United Nations (UN) Biodiversity Convention under its joint work programme on biodiversity and health with the World Health Organization (WHO). She has more than 17 years of experience as a sustainability professional working in policy evaluation and development, multi-stakeholder engagement, and interdisciplinary research with the UN, specialized agencies, the public and private sectors, and nongovernmental organizations. She has provided high-level scientific and policy advice in research and regulatory-compliance settings, primarily in the areas of biodiversity and ecosystem management and conservation, global and public health, One Health, climate change, and regulatory energy policy. She also jointly organized and led capacity-building workshops convened by the UN Biodiversity Convention and the World Health Organization (WHO), bringing together ministries of health and environment, experts, and local community representatives across more than 85 countries in Latin America, Africa, Europe, and the Association of Southeast Asian Nations region. She was a principal lead coordinating author of the WHO and Convention on Biological Diversity (CBD)-led *State of Knowledge Review, Connecting Global Priorities: Biodiversity and Human Health*, and has contributed to several other UN reports, most recently leading the development of biodiversity-inclusive policy guidance on One Health adopted at the 2018 UN Biodiversity Conference (COP 14). Prior to joining the CBD in 2010, she worked as a senior sustainability consultant focusing on sustainable development policy, energy regulation, and climate change, contributing to more than 35 energy regulatory proceedings across North America. She holds a master of science and a master of arts.

Danielle Sholly, Ph.D., M.S., is an animal scientist within the Office of New Animal Drug Evaluation at the U.S. Food and Drug Administration's Center for Veterinary Medicine (CVM). Dr. Sholly obtained her doctor of philosophy and master of science degrees in swine nutrition from Purdue University. Her graduate research focused on the impact of dietary modifications on animal growth and nutrient excretion from growing-finishing pigs. Dr. Sholly joined CVM in 2009 and enjoys the pre-approval side of new animal drug approval; reviewing target animal safety and effectiveness data for food animal drugs. She also enjoys collaborating on projects and issues that encompass the three branches of a One Health approach: human, animal, and environmental health.

Jonathan Sleeman, ECFVG, is currently the center director for the U.S. Geological Survey National Wildlife Health Center, where he leads a team of scientists and support staff to investigate and research wildlife diseases that threaten wildlife populations, public health, and the economy. He received his master's degree in zoology and his veterinary degree from the University of Cambridge and completed an internship and residency in zoological medicine at the University of Tennessee. He is a diplomate of the American College of Zoological Medicine. He has published widely on topics related to wildlife anesthesia, emerging diseases of wildlife, wildlife epidemiology, risk assessment, One Health, and Ecohealth. He holds a variety of leadership positions, including as a member of the World Organisation for Animal Health's Working Group on Wildlife, and is a board member for Ecohealth International. Current interests include development of national wildlife health programs in Asia and Africa, broad-scale wildlife disease risk assessments, and leadership skills in wildlife health.

Woutrina Smith, D.V.M., M.P.V.M., Ph.D., is a professor of infectious disease epidemiology in the School of Veterinary Medicine at the University of California, Davis (UC Davis), and co-leads the U.S. Agency for International Development (USAID) One Health Workforce–Next Generation Project working with AFROHUN and SEAOHUN. She also co-leads the multi-campus Planetary Health Center of Expertise within the UC Global Health Institute, and is an associate director at the UC Davis One Health Institute. Dr. Smith has worked on One Health research projects across Africa, Asia, and in the Americas, where multidisciplinary teams innovate together to solve complex health problems. Dr. Smith has received funding from diverse sources, including the National Institutes of Health, USAID, the U.S. Department of Defense, and the Bill & Melinda Gates Foundation to support her research and training programs.

Mark S. Smolinski, M.D., M.P.H., is the president of Ending Pandemics. He brings 25 years of experience in applying innovative solutions to improve disease prevention, response, and control across the globe. Dr. Smolinski is leading a well-knit team—bringing together technologists; human, animal, and environmental health experts; and key community stakeholders to co-create tools for early detection, advanced warning, and prevention of pandemic threats. Community health workers, village volunteers, farmers, and interested public citizens in Albania, Brazil, Cambodia, Europe, Laos, Myanmar, Tanzania, Thailand, and the United States are among those using their own solutions to address pressing local needs. Since 2009, Dr. Smolinski has served as the chief medical officer and director of Global Health at the Skoll Global Threats Fund (SGTF), where he developed the Ending Pandemics in Our Lifetime Initiative in 2012. His work at SGTF created a solid foundation for the work of Ending Pandemics, which branched out as an independent entity on January 1, 2018. Prior to SGTF, Dr. Smolinski developed the Predict and Prevent Initiative at Google.org, as part of the starting team at Google's philanthropic arm. Working with a team of engineers, Google Flu Trends (a project that had tremendous impact on the use of big data for disease surveillance) was created in partnership with the U.S. Centers for Disease Control and Prevention (CDC). Dr. Smolinski has served as vice president for biological programs at the Nuclear Threat Initiative (NTI), a public charity directed by CNN founder Ted Turner and former U.S. senator Sam Nunn. Before NTI, he led an 18-member expert committee of the Institute of Medicine on the 2003 landmark report *Microbial Threats to Health: Emergence, Detection, and Response*. Dr. Smolinski served as the sixth Luther Terry Fellow in Washington, DC, in the office of the U.S. surgeon general and as an epidemic intelligence officer with CDC. Dr. Smolinski received his B.S. in biology and M.D. from the University of Michigan in Ann Arbor. He is board certified in preventive medicine and public health and holds an M.P.H. from the University of Arizona, where he was recognized as the 2016 Alumnus of the Year. Dr. Smolinski was on the investigation team that discovered hantavirus, a newly identified pathogen, in 1993. His passion for helping all peoples of the world saves lives, improves livelihoods, and motivates partners.

Claire Standley, M.Sc., Ph.D., is an assistant research professor within Georgetown University's Center for Global Health Science and Security, with faculty appointments in the Department of Microbiology & Immunology and the Department of International Health. She is also affiliated with the Heidelberg Institute for Global Health in Heidelberg, Germany. Her research focuses on the analysis of health systems strengthening and international capacity building for public health, with an emphasis on multisectoral and integrated approaches for the prevention and control of infectious diseases, particularly in the context of public health emergency preparedness and response. Prior to joining Georgetown University, Dr. Standley was a senior research scientist at The George Washington University Milken Institute of Public Health, and also served as an American Association for the Advancement of Science science and technology policy fellow at the Department of State, where she supported programs for laboratory capacity building, disease surveillance, and cooperative health security research.

Dr. Standley received a B.A. (with honors) in natural sciences from the University of Cambridge, an M.Sc. in biodiversity, conservation, and management from the University of Oxford, and a Ph.D. in genetics (with a focus on biomedical parasitology) from the University of Nottingham, as part of a joint program with the Natural History Museum of London, and completed a postdoctoral fellowship in biodiversity and infectious diseases at Princeton University.

Rajeev Venkayya, M.D., is president of the Global Vaccine Business Unit at Takeda Pharmaceutical Company Ltd, where he leads a vertically integrated business developing vaccines for dengue, norovirus and Zika. He also oversees partnerships with the Japanese government to supply COVID-19 and pandemic influenza vaccines. He serves as an independent member of the board of the Coalition for Epidemic Preparedness Innovations (CEPI), which is funding and coordinating several vaccine development programs for severe acute respiratory syndrome coronavirus 2 (SARS-CoV-2). He is also on the board of the International AIDS Vaccine Initiative and is a life member of the Council on Foreign Relations.

Dr. Venkayya is currently co-leading Takeda's response to the COVID-19 outbreak, given his previous experience at the White House as special assistant to the president for biodefense. In this role, he was the principal author of the National Strategy for Pandemic Influenza (2005), and his office led the development and execution of the companion Implementation Plan (2006). His team conceived the strategy of early, coordinated implementation of non-pharmaceutical interventions to slow the spread of a pandemic virus, now known as "flattening the curve," that was described in the U.S. government's guidelines on community mitigation of pandemic influenza (2007). These guidelines were updated in 2017 to reflect the lessons of the 2009-H1N1 outbreak, and the concepts therein are being implemented or considered by governments around the world to slow the transmission of SARS-CoV-2.

Prior to joining Takeda, Dr. Venkayya served as director of vaccine delivery at the Bill & Melinda Gates Foundation's Global Health Program, where he was responsible for the foundation's top two priorities of polio eradication and the introduction of new vaccines into developing countries through Gavi, the Vaccine Alliance. He also served on the board of Gavi.

Dr. Venkayya trained in pulmonary and critical care medicine at the University of California, San Francisco, where he also served on the faculty. He was a resident and chief medical resident in internal medicine at the University of Michigan. He received his B.S./M.D. from the Northeast Ohio Universities College of Medicine, where he was inducted into the Alpha Omega Alpha honorary medical society.

Supaporn Wacharapluesadee, Ph.D., is the laboratory head at the Thai Red Cross Emerging Infectious Diseases Health Science Centre (TRC-EID), King Chulalongkorn Memorial Hospital, Faculty of Medicine, Chulalongkorn University, a World Health Organization (WHO) Collaborating Centre for Research and Training on Viral Zoonoses. Her research interests include emerging infectious diseases in bats (including Nipah, rabies, coronavirus, and novel pathogens) as well as molecular diagnoses and sequencing of viruses. TRC-EID is responsible for molecular diagnoses services to the hospital, and is the reference laboratory for rabies virus, Middle East respiratory syndrome coronavirus, Ebola, Zika, and other infectious disease diagnoses for the Ministry of Public Health, Thailand. She has served and consulted on several WHO and Thai government committees. Dr. Wachaeapluesadee's team was the first to positively identify a human COVID-19 infection outside China.

Michael Wilkes, M.D., M.P.H., Ph.D., is widely known for his efforts to introduce medical students to the humanistic side of being a physician, and for working tirelessly to include the public health and social sciences as part of training physicians. During his tenure as vice dean of the medical school he led the way toward enormous changes in medical education at the University of California, Davis (UC Davis), including the rural prime program, the college system of mentoring, and a dramatic shift away from lectures toward small group and interactive learning. Dr. Wilkes introduced UC Davis's "Doctoring" curriculum, a series of classes and seminars for all four years of medical school. Topics within the curriculum include One Health, interprofessional education, leadership, doctor–patient communication, and clinical reasoning to name but a few. Dr. Wilkes has extensive experience in the development, management, and evaluation of eLearning technologies. In his current capacity as director of global health he works locally with the UC Davis veterinary and nursing faculty and with medical and health sciences schools around the world, helping to build capacity by creating environments to train the most capable health providers to address local health needs. He serves as a reviewer for many medical publications and is an award-winning journalist currently with National Public Radio. He is also an adolescent health physician.

Dana Wiltz-Beckham, D.V.M., M.P.H., M.B.A., earned her undergraduate degree from Prairie View A&M University, her doctor of veterinary medicine degree from Tuskegee University, and her M.P.H./M.B.A. from Benedictine University. After veterinary medical school, Dr. Wiltz-Beckham worked in The Gambia, West Africa, as a veterinarian and laboratory diagnostician for one year. Returning to the United States, she trained at the University of Texas Southwestern Medical Center as a National Institutes of Health fellow in comparative medicine. Dr. Wiltz-Beckham has more than 20 years of experience in the public health and research fields. Her professional background consists of jobs as a laboratory animal veterinary consultant; director of the Palo Alto College Veterinary Technology Program in San Antonio, Texas; Regional Zoonosis Control Veterinarian for the Texas Department of Health HSR 6/5S; and director of Animal Services, chief epidemiologist, and director of Community Health Services for Galveston County Health District. Currently, she serves as the director for the Office of Science, Surveillance, and Technology at Harris County Public Health. Additionally, she is a long-standing adjunct faculty member at the University of Texas Medical Branch. Dr. Wiltz-Beckham has worked extensively within the Southeast region of Texas on disease investigation, One Health initiatives, emergency management, education, and surveillance.

Irene Xagoraraki, Ph.D., is an associate professor of environmental engineering at Michigan State University. She earned her Ph.D. and M.S. degrees in environmental engineering from the University of Wisconsin–Madison and her B.S. degree in environmental science from the University of the Aegean in Greece. Her research is focused on water quality engineering emphasizing protection of public health and prevention of waterborne disease. She is interested in microbial contaminants and their fate in water systems. Her current research focuses on viral outbreak identification and prediction using wastewater-based epidemiology. Her research projects have been funded by the National Science Foundation, the Michigan Department of Environment, Great Lakes and Energy, the Great Lakes Water Authority, the Environmental Protection Agency, the Department of Homeland Security, Water Research Foundation, Water Environmental Research Foundation, and other agencies.